# GEO-ECOLOGY OF MALNUTRITION

# *GEO-ECOLOGY OF MALNUTRITION*

## *A Study of the Haryana Children*

SURINDER K. AGGARWAL

INTER-INDIA PUBLICATIONS
D-17 RAJA GARDEN EXTN. NEW DELHI-110015 (INDIA)

**Cataloging in Publication Data—DK**

Aggarwal, Surinder K., 1943-

Geo-ecology of malnutrition.

Bibliography: p.

Includes index.

1. Malnutrition in children—India—Haryana. 2. Nutrition disorders in children—India—Haryana. 3. Children—India—Haryana—Nutrition. 4. Medical geography—India—Haryana. I. Title.

ISBN 81-210-0074-2

First Published in India in 1986

Surinder K. **Aggarwal** (*b. 1943-* )

Published in India by:
M.C. Mittal
INTER-INDIA PUBLICATIONS
D-17, RAJA GARDEN EXTN.,
NEW DELHI-110015 (INDIA)
PHONE : 5413145

*Printed in India by*
Alka Enterprises
*at* Sunil Printers, Naraina, New Delhi-110028

# Foreword

By its very nature the problem of pediatric nutrition is significant throughout the world, but it is of vital importance in the Developing World where most of the world's children live but unhappily struggle to survive under conditions of mal and under-nourishment. Since the problem of child nutrition is very complex, its study cannot be confined only to the medical and health professions. These professions cannot be expected to uncover all the causes of under-nourishment which lie within the social, cultural and economic contexts of the society, let alone providing adequate solutions. The importance of Dr. Aggarwal's work lies in its serious attempt to unravel the problem of child nutrition within its socio-economic milieu yet at the scale of the individual child.

In a systematic and scientifically rigorous manner, Dr. Aggarwal has examined child nutrition in ten purposely selected villages of Haryana by taking a sample of over three hundred children between the ages of six and thirty-six months. Dr. Aggarwal has combined relevant analytical methodology by use of descriptive and multivariate statistics with the commitment of a concerned scholar to produce a study which reflects both objectivity and a keen desire to see a healthier new generation. Having known the author for several years, especially during the progress of this work in the United States, I have been greatly impressed with the simple minded devotion and a rather substantial financial sacrifice he underwent to carry out his field work in India. Dr. Aggarwal has, in fact, set a worthy example for young scholars by demonstrating that personal field work and on site observations are necessary for good applied geography research. The tendency among many researchers to favor the chair and the computer in place of personal field observations can prove dangerous in the long run. No amount of mailed questionnaire surveys and fast data processing alone can come to grips with the intricate problem of child malnutrition, so prevalent among the rural poor and illiterate families. The relevance of Dr. Aggarwal's work is, happily, not confined to one discipline either through its conceptualization or analysis although it highlights the often neglected spatial dimension of malnutrition.

Dr. Aggarwal's study shows that although pediatric malnutrition on the whole is not as widespread in the agriculturally progressive Haryana as in several other parts of India, but the variations in malnutrition are nevertheless substantial from village to village and from one caste group to the other. Agrarian prosperity has not necessarily resulted in a commensurately better nutritional status of the poorest segment of the society. An important implication of Dr. Aggarwal's finding is that increased agricultural productivity should not lull us to neglect the very real but often masked problem of child malnutrition among the very poor families. In addition, Dr. Aggarwal has amply demonstrated that improved environmental sanitation and adoption of family planning are positively associated with better child nutrition. The former reducing the chance of infection (especially diarrhea and consequent dehydration) and the latter improving the dietary intake of infants and young children.

A major strength of the methodology utilized in Dr. Aggarwal's work is that target groups for nutritional intervention can be and have been identified. Surely, this can be very useful for planning officials when developing strategies for improving child health status in the rural areas within the constraints of scarce resources. Thus, the holistic perspective adopted in this book should make it valuable not only to researchers in the social sciences but also to the health professionals and especially the agencies concerned with delivering maternal and child health programs.

I fervently hope that young social scientists, especially medical geographers will take up the national and intellectual task of addressing the problem of child nutrition throughout India. This is the challenge presented by Dr. Aggarwal's work focused on one of the more prosperous regions of India. What are the dimensions of child malnutrition in other parts of India?

Are the determinants of child malnutrition the same in different regions of India? Are the contrasts between different ecological zones indeed significant? These and numerous other questions are not merely of intellectual import but concern the very future of India. I certainly feel privileged to have been asked to write this foreword.

SURINDER M. BHARDWAJ
Professor of Geography
Kent State University
Kent, Ohio, U.S.A.

# Acknowledgements

Most research works owe gratitude to several individuals and institutions at different stages of their initiation, progress, and completion. This study is no exception. First and foremost I owe a special gratitude to Professor Surinder M. Bhardwaj, who aroused interest in me in the growing field of Medical Geography and particularly on a surmounting problem of "malnutrition" within developing countries. He has been a constant source of inspiration, encouragement and optimism at different stages of the completion of this research. My gratitude also goes to Professor Milton E. Harvey, Professor Gordon A. Hodgkins, and Professor Charles F. Kegley for their valuable suggestions and constructive criticism. I am thankful to Prof. A.B. Mukerji of Panjab University, Chandigarh, for his constant inspiration to get this work published.

My thanks goes to the Geography Department at Kent State University in granting the University Fellowship and a travel grant from the Beck Fund of the Geography Department in conducting field work in India. While in India, the help of several individuals at the state, district and village levels and of several institutions is acknowledged in organisation, administration and operationalisation of the study. The families of the surveyed villages were generous in hospitality and enthusiastic about the study. Their enthusiasm was reflected by the fact that most families wanted to be part of the survey. Their endeavor is deeply appreciated. The field work was a real experience to the author in not only generating the field data rather than gaining the insights of the malnutrition problem embedded in the quality of life and other life parameters.

Several other individuals deserve special thanks who provided help in different capacities. Kind hospitality of Mohan and Vijaya Shreshtha and Prem and Uma Gupta is deeply appreciated in providing me comfort and home environment while my family was away to India. My special thanks goes to my wife, Surmesh, who not only typed several drafts of this work, but also has been a constant source of inspiration and moral support through the progress of this study. My thanks to Mr. Krishan Kumar and Bachi Ram of University of Delhi for their technical help in the cartographic work of the book. Finally, I dedicate this study to the children of Haryana, who provided me an opportunity in understanding the iceberg nature of the malnutrition problem.

It may be mentioned to the readers that American spellings are used in this book due to the progress of this work in the United States.

Delhi SURINDER K. AGGARWAL
April 6, 1986

# Contents

# List of Figures

# List of Tables

# List of Illustrations

# 1

# Introduction

THE malnutrition[1] problem is of great concern in the developing countries because of its mass prevalence, its tragic human implications, and its adverse impact on economic development processes. The magnitude of the problem suggests a need for rigorous effort in estimating its prevalence, specific causes, and feasible solutions. Until relatively recently, nutrition and other aspects of health have been considered to be the concern of the medical profession. Increasingly, however, social and behavioral scientists have begun to make their contribution and the various preventive dimensions of health care are being examined. Realizing that malnutrition, particularly protein calorie malnutrition (hereafter referred to simply as PCM), is the overriding health problem of most developing countries, the present study is an attempt to:

(*i*) Estimate the prevalence of PCM in the young children (6-36 months) of rural Haryana,
(*ii*) Identify the determinants which most influence the nutritional status of the young children, and
(*iii*) Suggest planned interventions for the target groups based on derived critical factors.

The major thrust of the study, however, hinges on the first two objectives. In order to arrive at the above objectives, the following scheme will be followed:

## Prevalence of PCM

The prevalence of PCM in the sampled children will be assessed using weight for age parameter (Jelliffe's scheme of PCM classification[2]). This is the most common anthropometric measure suitable for field conditions. A detailed discussion on the choice and appropriateness of different methods of assessing nutritional status (N.S.) is given in Chapter 4. The prevalence of PCM will be assessed for different locations, age-groups, and major socio-economic group children such that target populations or areas could be identified. This seems to be the first step in estimating and planning for correcting the malnutrition problem in a community.

## The Determinants of PCM

The second step in correcting the malnutrition problems involves the identification of the correlates which most influence the N.S. Two issues seem crucial in identifying the causative factors: conceptual and methodological.

The conceptual part will tell us how the causative factors of malnutrition are interrelated with each other. This is treated at length in the conceptualization chapter. A geo-ecological[3] approach is pursued in this effort. According to the ecological component of this approach, the N.S. of a community is (supposedly) influenced by a complex interaction involving food availability, income, environmental conditions, personal hygiene, education, size of a family, and several other interrelated factors. The geographical (geo) component will add to our understanding of the causative factors varying from place to place. Together, the components of the geo-ecological approach, therefore, provide us with a holistic treatment of the malnutrition problem. It is clear that unless the answers to the diseases are sought within the context in which they occur, we shall not be able to plan for effective control, prevention, and ultimately elimination. It is at this point that the geographical approach becomes important. It may be added that the eco-system perspective has also been suggested by Stoddart and many other geographers to help explain the complex relationships of geographical sub-systems.[4] Among the nutrition experts, Patwardhan and Pollack[5] have strongly stressed the consideration of geographical factors in identification and assessment of deficiency diseases. It is true that J.M. May's studies provided the ecological dimensions in human malnutrition,[6] but the scale of his studies (continental/country) and the paucity of uniform data at that level mitigate an indepth analysis. The present study, by concentrating on a small geographic area of India and by generating more rigorous data, will try to fill such a gap.

Methodologically, little research is noticed where myriad factors of malnutrition have been subjected to rigorous quantitative analysis. Levison's study on Morinda children of Punjab, India, is the only study known to the author which has tried to isolate the economic determinants of malnutrition using multivariate techniques.[7] In the present study, multiple classification analysis[8] (MCA), from the battery of multivariate methods, has been utilized in estimating the relationships of possible determinants with the N.S. This model shows an advantage over several similar multivariate techniques. It can treat the mixed modes of data and can estimate the combined and category influence of each interrelated variable. In this way we can identify the critical category children who need planned intervention for correcting the malnutrition problem. The utility of this model over other models is elaborated on in Chapter 4. The application of this method in estimating the relationship of causative factors with N.S. is given in Chapter 6.

**Solutions of Malnutrition**

The third component of the research pertains to solutions of malnutrition. The intent of this section is to present not a planning strategy but rather the approach that the identified critical factors should be the basis of resource allocation for combating malnutrition.

The geo-ecological approach, by identifying the critical factors in different areas, would suggest the most realistic and efficient way to utilize the scarce funds and expertise for the specific intervention. In the earlier studies, blanket intervention strategies are suggested with little concern for relative contribution of the causative factors.

In summary, the geo-ecological approach is suggested in the present study on Haryana because of:

(*i*) A variety of milieu in Haryana,
(*ii*) The holistic conceptualization of the problem, and
(*iii*) Utility in the planning process.

Briefly, the contents of this research take the following form:

— Chapter 2 is a typological literature review on the malnutrition problem in India as discussed from the perspective of prevalence, causes, and solutions.
— The ecological conceptual framework of the PCM problem is presented in Chapter 3.
— Research design and methodological issues pertaining to assessment of nutritional status, and use of MCA model in identifying the causes of PCM are discussed in Chapter 4.
— In Chapter 5 is presented the initial assessment of the nutrition problem in Haryana children based on the survey data.
— Chapter 6 basically discusses the specific determinants of PCM in the sampled children as estimated by MCA model.
— Chapter 7 presents the summary of conclusions and planning suggestions.

## REFERENCES

1. The term malnutrition in this study is used interchangeably with PCM. In nutrition literature, little distinction is made between the two while addressing the general malnutrition problem. In the present study, however, we are concerned with Protein-Calorie-Malnutrition (PCM), as it is the overriding problem among young children.
2. For a detailed discussion on the scheme and its basis of classification see D.B. Jelliffe, *The Assessment of the Nutritional Status of the Community* (Geneva: World Health Organization, 1966).
3. A geo-ecological approach simply means to explore how several causative factors of malnutrition are interrelated, and vary from area to area.
4. Stoddart, D. R., "Geography and the Ecological Approach," *Geography* 50 (1965), 242-51.

5. Patwardhan, V. N., "Geographic Distribution of Malnutrition," *Proceedings of the Seventh International Congress of Nutrition*, Vol. 1 (Toronto: Pergamon Press, 1966), pp. 27-33; Herbert Pollack, *Proceedings of the Seventh International Congress*, 1: 362-70.
6. May, Jacques M., *The Ecology of Human Disease* (New York: M.D. Publications Inc., 1958).
7. Levison, F. James, *Morinda: An Economic Analysis of Malnutrition Among Young Children in Rural India*, Cornell-MIT International Nutrition Policy Series, Vol. 1 (Cambridge, Mass : MIT Press, 1974).
8. Andrews, Frank M., *et al.*, *Multiple Classification Analysis* (Ann Arbor, Michigan: The University of Michigan, 1975).

# 2

# Perspectives on the Malnutrition Problem in India

## Introduction

THE malnutrition problem in India has been well recognized, although its exact estimate, solutions, and implications were obscure until recently. In 1943, the Bhore committee had roughly estimated the severity of this problem in India.[1] Inadequate nutrition was stated explicitly as one of the major factors in high infant mortality and the health.[2] On the recommendation of the committee, the Government of India did allocate substantial funds for improving health, but nutrition did not receive direct attention. Nutrition was included under water supply and sanitation. Even after the Independence of India, nutrition received scant attention until the Fifth Five Year Plan. It is only in this plan that a section is devoted exclusively to nutrition and a substantial outlay of 405 million rupees ($50 million) is allocated to nutrition programs.[3] The current outlay, amounting to only 1.1 per cent of the total outlay of the Fifth Five Year Plan[4] may seem inadequate to solve the problem. However, the direct concern is a notable step in the right direction. A comprehensive approach, by integrating the existing feeding programs with immunization, improvement in environmental sanitation, and family welfare planning, is suggested to ameliorate the problem. Notwithstanding the benefits of this approach, the implementation is still in the embryonic stage. A coordination between the States and the Central Government is strongly desired for the effective implementation of such programs. In short, one can say that India is pursuing the nutrition problem with a serious concern.

In developing a national concern, the research effort in different but allied disciplines of nutrition science, biochemistry, physiological anthropology, home science and pediatrics cannot be minimized. In general, the thrust of such studies seems to remain the estimations of nutritional status of the vulnerable groups, through biochemical, clinical, and anthropometric measures. Special mention may be made of the National Institute of Nutrition (formerly, Nutrition Research Laboratories) where intensive research is being done on human multifaceted aspects of nutrition with a national interest. The institute has conducted nation-wide food consumption and anthropometric surveys to estimate the malnutrition problem in India. The results have been presented in the Diet Atlas of India[5] and Nutrition Atlas of India.[6]

The studies on prevalence and etiology of malnutrition have been carried out quite extensively. Presently, the nutrition experts have begun to realize that the nutrition studies should not end only in identifying the etiology; rather, ecological studies should be pursued to identify, precisely, the socio-economic-cultural constraints of the malnutrition problem, so that practical measures can be implemented.

The theoretical basis for relating malnutrition or under-nutrition with ecological factors is well documented.[7] However, precise estimates of ecological determinants, with a comparative analysis for different geographic areas, are still lacking.

In order to formulate some firm basis for further research, a critical review of some earlier works, their findings, approaches, and shortcomings, is presented in the following discussion. In view of the objectives of the present research, only studies related to assessment, causative factors, and solutions of malnutrition problem are examined here.

## MAJOR FINDINGS OF NUTRITION STUDIES DONE ON INDIA

### General Nature of the Malnutrition Problem

Based on direct and indirect methods of assessment,[8] the prevalence of PCM has been identified as the most important and widespread nutrition problem in India.[9] Young children below 5 years of age, from low income social groups and from rural and urban areas, are noted to be suffering from some degree of PCM.[10] Chatterjee estimates that the prevalence of PCM in children 1-5 years of age is around 2 per cent showing frank deficiency, and 85 per cent showing a relatively milder form of deficiency (around 70-90 per cent of standard weight[11]) in the form of Kwashirkor and Marasmus. He also estimates that nearly a million children die every year due to PCM.[12]

Several other studies have also identified a synergistic relationship between PCM and the incidence of several infections and non-nutritional diseases.[13] Therefore, PCM along with other diseases has been found to be an affliction of most young children in low socio-economic groups. Children from middle and higher income groups are also stated to be suffering from PCM; however, the intensity and prevalence is comparatively low in these groups.

## STUDIES RELATED TO NUTRITIONAL ASSESSMENT

### Food Consumption Studies

The calorie intake and the quality and quantity of nutrient intake in an individual can be precisely measured by the food consumption levels. Because of this fact, food consumption levels of different biological and socio-economic groups at community, local, regional, and national level have been assessed through food consumption surveys, diet surveys, and food balance sheets. At this point only those studies are mentioned which are extensive in scale and are of national importance. The most important study at the national level was conducted by the Indian Council of Medical Research for a period covering 1960 through 1969. The food consumption pattern for different states as revealed by this study, is shown in Table 2.1. Since no current study could be available on food consumption pattern, the conditions might be different at present.

Table 2.1 shows that except for cereals, most other foods fall below the recommended daily allowance (RDA) in most of the states. Pulses, milk, and milk products, and other animal foods

TABLE 2.1 : **Food Consumption Pattern in Different States of India (1960-69)**

(*Grams per person per day*)

| State* | Number of surveys | Rice | Wheat | Millets and other cereals | Total cereals | Pulses | Leafy vegetables | Other vegetables | Fruits | Fats and oils | Milk & milk products | Meat, fish and egg | Sugar and jaggery |
|---|---|---|---|---|---|---|---|---|---|---|---|---|---|
| Andhra Pradesh | 111 | 335 | 10 | 121 | 466 | 29 | 34 | 34 | 1 | 11 | 65 | 11 | 9 |
| Bihar | 62 | 267 | 97 | 89 | 453 | 42 | 21 | 69 | 3 | 8 | 20 | 8 | 5 |
| Gujarat | 1 | 73 | 13 | 339 | 425 | 43 | 26 | 49 | — | 5 | 7 | 6 | 6 |
| Jammu and Kashmir | 3 | 212 | 18 | 359 | 589 | 8 | 163 | 63 | — | 10 | 14 | 3 | 12 |
| Kerala | 37 | 296 | 38 | 7 | 341 | 24 | 8 | 170 | 36 | 7 | 52 | 52 | 18 |
| Madhya Pradesh | 2 | 37 | 356 | 259 | 652 | 55 | 4 | 41 | 86 | 19 | 138 | 11 | 38 |
| Maharashtra | 9 | 241 | 61 | 196 | 498 | 33 | 17 | 62 | 9 | 15 | 49 | 27 | 31 |
| Mysore | 45 | — | — | — | 607 | 26 | 9 | 19 | 1 | 2 | 56 | 3 | — |
| Punjab and Haryana | 22 | 42 | 378 | 99 | 519 | 35 | 44 | 93 | 13 | 17 | 317 | 7 | 97 |
| Rajasthan | 31 | 8 | 183 | 266 | 457 | 43 | 10 | 30 | 1 | 34 | 94 | 2 | 16 |
| Tamilnadu | 114 | 288 | 11 | 57 | 356 | 16 | 8 | 52 | 5 | 6 | 26 | 13 | 6 |
| Uttar Pradesh | 113 | 161 | 154 | 133 | 448 | 55 | 38 | 97 | 21 | 16 | 91 | 8 | 32 |
| West Bengal | 24 | 336 | 86 | — | 422 | 30 | 51 | 112 | 3 | 17 | 52 | 30 | 22 |
| All India | 574 | 241 | 84 | 109 | 434 | 34 | 21 | 71 | 10 | 12 | 69 | 14 | 19 |
| Suggested Allowances for a typical balanced diet | — | — | — | — | 370 | 70 | 110 | 125 | 37 | 38 | 180 | 35 | 40 |

*Source*: C. Gopalan *et al*., *Diet Atlas of India* (Hyderabad: National Institute of Nutrition, 1971), 118.

*Data about all States not available.

fall below the recommended daily allowance (RDA) in most of the states. Pulses, milk, and milk products, and other animal foods, the major sources of protein, are lacking in most states. In the consumption of milk and milk products, only the states of Punjab and Haryana (317 gms) exceed the recommended allowance of 180 gms. per person per day. Madhya Pradesh and Rajasthan are somewhat closer, but all other states show far less consumption of milk, a very important source of quality protein and several minerals and vitamins. Similarly, consumption of meat, fish, and eggs is far less than the recommended allowance. Pulses (legumes) which form the major source of vegetable protein in Indian diet are found somewhat closer to the recommended allowance of 70 gms. per day. In most southern states consumption of pulses is relatively small in comparison to the northern and central states. Cereals, the major source of calories and to a lesser degree of proteins in Indian diet, are consumed above the recommended allowance (Table 2.1). The greatest deficiency in the food pattern is apparent for vegetables, fruits, vegetable oils and animal fats. Such inadequacies in the Indian diet have been generally associated with deficiencies of vitamin A, iron, and calories. The general sufficiency in cereals and deficiency in pulses and animal products may allude to the shortage of calories and especially lack of protein in the Indian diet. Variations in the nutritional status of urban and rural populations are also explained by the differences in the dietary pattern of the respective populations. Such differences are explained not only because of variations in income, but also due to micro-environmental conditions, variety in food, prices of food, attitudes toward certain foods, and size of the family. No single factor is completely responsible for such variations. Rather an additive effect of all such factors in an urban milieu generates more dismal ecological conditions for malnutrition.

Sukhatme, on the basis of his Maharashtra study, concludes that urban diets differ from rural diets in two respects: (*i*) their total energy and protein contents are smaller, but (*ii*) they are more varied in composition.[14] In this study, he analyzes that urban diets have a 46 per cent deficit in calories, and 41 per cent deficit in proteins, whereas rural diets, in the same order, have 26 per cent and 22 per cent deficit.[15] Even with such a significant variation, Sukhatme purports that protein deficiency in urban areas is not as extensive as it appears. He argues that the urban diets contain more variety, and, therefore, the proportion of utilizable protein in the diet is likely to be larger than in the rural diet to compensate in part for its lower protein intake. Rao and others observed higher prevalence rates of different nutritional deficiency signs in urban slum children as compared to their rural counterparts.[16]

They also observed that the diets of urban children were relatively deficient in protein and caloric centents, which supports Sakhatme's observations. Indirectly, such differences can also be compared through total food expenditure as per cent of total monthly expenditure. In general, the rural areas are stated to stand higher than urban areas in their per cent of expenditure on food.[17] Although the rural/urban variation in nutritional status is mentioned by such studies, the causes for such differentiation need further exploration.

At a regional level, Gopalan and Rao have found a high deficiency of calories and moderate deficiency of proteins in young children for five regions in India.[18] According to their analysis, based on the standardized dietary survey, Delhi and Poona children were comparatively higher in protein and calorie intake than their counterparts in Bombay, Vellore, and Hyderabad regions. Based on food consumption levels, several deficiency diseases are analysed by Husain and Khan for the western region of Uttar Pradesh.[19] Blyn has recently reported declining mean nutritional adequacy rations for Punjab and Haryana cultivators' families during the 1950-51 to 1968-69 period.[20]

Village level micro studies have also been carried out by several individuals, agencies, and state governments. An annotated bibliography of such studies has been compiled by the Institute of Development Studies, University of Sussex.[21] A perusal of the monograph divulges interregional and intraregional deficiencies in the intake of various nutrients (primarily vitamin A, vitamin C, and riboflavin, as well as calories). For example, in an intensive comparative study on children in selected villages of Punjab (Narangwal Rural Health Research Center) the following findings were reported in the monograph:[22]

> A program of nutritional supplementation with and without medical care for children (0-3 years) produced

(*i*) a moderate improvement in nutritional status; (*ii*) significantly lowered mortality rates in children 12-35 months, and significantly improved haemoglobin levels. The beneficial effects were greater in children over 12 months of age. The medical care program seemed to have little or no additional benefit beyond that produced by nutrition alone.

**Anthropometric Studies**

Such studies seem to be conducted more often than the food consumption studies because of their ease and comparative validity. Relationships between weights, heights, age, arm circumference, head circumference, skinfold thickness, and other somatic parameters have been extensively used to measure the nutritional status. On the basis of least cost balance diets proposed by the Indian Council of Medical Research, the prevailing extent of malnutrition in India was assessed in a nationwide nutrition survey for pre-school children.[23] Classified according to weight deficit for age, 18 per cent of the children were suffering from Grade III malnutrition, 65 per cent from Grade II, and 14 per cent from Grade I malnutrition.[24]

Regional variations in several anthropometric measure on young children are clearly discernible in the Nutrition Atlas of India.[25] For example, average birth weights of children in poor families are highest in Punjab (2899 gms) and Delhi (3100 gms); moderate in the southern states of Andhra (2731 gms) and Tamilnadu (2778 gms); lowest in eastern states of Bihar (2714 gms) and West Bengal (2640 gms). Significant differences in birth weight are noticed in poor and wealthy families for all states of India. Similar interregional and intraregional differences on somatic parameters of young children are perceptible by comparing many other studies.[26]

In assessing the nutritional status, the above works clearly indicate mass prevalence of malnutrition among pre-school children from low income groups. Regional and socio-economic contrasts are also noticed in most such studies.

## FACTORS INFLUENCING MALNUTRITION

Factors influencing nutritional status have been extensively investigated both empirically and theoretically. Broadly, these can be grouped as etiological and geographical. The former are more immediate and can be labelled as causative, whereas the latter are remote and are termed as influencing factors. In most Indian studies, the empirical positive relationship between the malnutrition state of young children and etiological factors such as infectious diseases, gastrointestinal diseases, defective food intake (in terms of quality, quantity and time), congenital defects, and malabsorption has been well established.[27] On the other hand, the geographical factors such as physical environment,[28] demographic variables,[29] and socio-economic and cultural[30] factors are stated to have bearing upon the availability and consumption of food. These factors individually prohibit the consumption of such foods.[31] An interesting example of food habits (food faddism) was noticed during the early Green Revolution in India and Pakistan. The new high yielding varieties of wheat (Mexican Dwarfs) were not consumed in some cultural groups due to color, taste, and the fear that the *chapatis* (unleavened bread) made of new seeds will make men impotent. Presenting urban and rural contrasts in food habits, Ghai observes that prolonged breast-feeding in rural areas prohibits the child from getting adequate calories, and thereby precipitates PCM.[32] He contends that general poverty and unsanitary conditions in the rural areas discourage the use of early weaning foods (the major source of calories). Since many mothers have poor health, breast-feeding alone is not sufficient to provide all the nutritional needs of the child. Consequently, children who are breast-fed exclusively for prolonged periods are usually malnourished. In the urban areas, he maintains early weaning is more often practised in well-to-do families or by working mothers. Weaning practices are generally satisfactory. The standard of hygiene is better and, therefore, early weaning helps in improving the nutritional status. Faulty food habits related to taboos (such as cold and hot foods[33]), religious foods, super foods, and ceremonial foods are attached to the selection, preparation and intake of foods. Food avoidances, and preferences of this nature, restrict the intake of a variety of foods and, therefore, exacerbate the deficiency diseases.

Economic factors are also highly associated with nutritional status. Quoting Gopalan, Chakravarti indicates that economic condition is a very significant factor in determining not only the amounts of non-vegetarian foods consumed but also the practice of non-vegetarianism, since most people of low income groups are perhaps vegetarian because of economic necessity.[34] Levinson in his Morinda study observes that among the Ramadasias (scheduled castes, usually landless agricultural labour) the factor most critically inhibiting improvement in their nutritional status is income.[35] Health contrasts reflected in parameters such as weight, height, arm and head circumference are also reported in several micro studies for different income groups in rural and urban areas of India.

## SOLUTIONS OF THE MALNUTRITION PROBLEM

There are several studies oriented toward specific or general solutions of the malnutrition problem in India. A careful review of available literature on nutrition planning suggests two kinds of approaches/strategies. The empirical studies, as mentioned earlier, have suggested solutions based on the identified immediate causes. The most identified causes are faulty food habits, poverty, large size of the family, high infant mortality, infections and other diseases, and defective food intake. Most often these causes are identified independent of the other associated causes. This fact makes these studies purely descriptive rather than analytical in scientific terms. Elimination or mitigation of such causes has been suggested as the feasible solution to combat malnutrition in the most vulnerable groups. To implement the suggestions, programs oriented to nutrition education, family planning, maternal and child welfare, fortification and supplementation of children's food, and augmenting food production are generally recommended.[36]

On the other hand, solutions are also being proposed in a more conceptual and analytical framework. With a comprehensive outlook, alternative integrated intervention strategies, and more recently, analytical approaches within an ecological and systems framework are being considered seriously by the nutrition planners and the government. Operation research methods, *e.g.*, cost benefit analysis, linear programing, input-output analysis, and systems analysis, are being applied to analyze the outcome of the intervention inputs. In India's

Fourth Five Year Plan, linear programing was used to determine least cost patterns of increasing total food supplies to meet nutrient intake deficits.[37] A systems approach was used in the state of Tamilnadu for identifying causes and solutions for nutrition planning based on exclusive systems philosophy. This approach is regarded as a conceptual approach, a holistic way of looking at a problem to sharpen the decision-making process.

The Government of India has initiated several Applied Nutrition Programs (ANP), primarily after the harsh experience of periodic crop failures resulting in mass food shortages in several parts of India. As many as forty schemes were implemented during the Fourth Five Year Plan and are proposed to be intensified during the Fifth Five Year Plan.[38] The schemes included in the Nutrition Sector in the Fourth and Fifth Five Year Plans are broadly grouped under the following headings:

(*i*) Supplementary Feeding Programs,
(*ii*) Production, Processing and Supply Schemes,
(*iii*) Programs relating to nutrition education, and
(*iv*) Health-based Nutrition Schemes.

An excellent critical review of such programs in India and elsewhere is given by Berg.[39] Based on Berg's analysis, some of the lessons which can be learned from the Indian experiment on nutrition planning are: (*i*) the scale of thinking at the national level is quite large, (*ii*) programs do not develop according to a predetermined master plan, (*iii*) bureaucratic principles can be overcome if commitment is strong, (*iv*) much of the buoyancy is produced by a constellation of enlightened businessmen and scientists rather than politicians, (*v*) sophisticated food technology can be applied beyond conventional boundaries of food habits, (*vi*) a system approach is better than the conventional approaches, and (*vii*) political attractiveness is essential in the nutrition programs. In addition to the above lessons and hiatuses, an area level approach in nutrition planning seems lacking.

The findings of the above studies reveal various attributes of the malnutrition problem in India. However, to get a comprehensive understanding, to unravel new areas of research, and to broaden the conceptualization, an appraisal of some gaps in the nutrition research on India seems essential. Based on the above literature review some lacunae are summarized below.

**Limitations of Previous Nutrition Studies**

From a social scientist and particularly geographic perspective, the following limitations were observed after perusal of the previous studies:

(*i*) A paucity of ecological conceptualization of the nutrition problem,
(*ii*) General imprecision with estimation of the determinants of nutritional status,
(*iii*) Lack of a spatial comparative approach in the analysis of the nutrition problem and also nutrition planning, and
(*iv*) Lack of concensus on precise measurement of nutritional status based on prevalent clinical or anthropometric parameters.

It may be made clear that these are not the only gaps needing attention. These may vary from one researcher to the other, depending on his disciplinary background and purpose of the study. However, from a geographic perspective these limitations have been observed by the author in the nutrition literature examined. The present study is an attempt to fill some of the above deficiencies in the now growing field of medical geography.

REFERENCES

1. Reported in Government of India, *Report of the Health Survey and Planning Committee* (New Delhi: Government of India Press, 1962).
2. *Ibid.*, p. 15.
3. Government of India, *Draft Fifth Five Year Plan: 1974-79*, Vol. 1 (New Delhi: Government of India Press, 1973), p. 246.
4. *Plan: 1974-79*, Vol. 2 (New Delhi: Government of India Press, 1973), p. 83.

5. Gopalan, C., *et al.*, *Diet Atlas of India* (Hyderabad: National Institute of Nutrition, 1971).
6. Gopalan, C. and Vijaya Raghavan, *Nutrition Atlas of India* (Hyderabad: National Institute of Nutrition, Indian Council of Medical Research, 1971).
7. See for example Paul Gyorgy and O.L. Kline, ed., *Malnutrition is a Problem of Ecology* (New York: Karger, 1970).
8. Direct methods include food consumption patterns, anthropometric measurements, clinical signs, and biochemical levels. Infant mortality and general morbidity patterns of the young children are usually considered the indirect methods of assessment.
9. Gopalan, C., *Proceedings of the First Asian Congress on Nutrition*, Hyderabad, India, 1972.
10. Among several studies of this nature, special mention may be made to:

    Banik, N.D., *et al.*, "A Longitudinal Study of Protein Calorie Malnutrition in North Indian Pre-School Children," *Indian Journal of Pediatric* 38 (1971): 147-52; S.M. Pereria, Growth and Development of Children in Under Previleged Communities, Tamilnadu," *Indian Journal of Medical Research* 59 (June 1971); 164-76; F. James Levinson, *Morinda: An Economic Analysis of Malnutrition*; J.S. Mathur *et al.*, "Nutritional Disorders Among Children Below 5 years in a Rural Community," *Indian Journal of Pediatrics* 41 (1974), 185-91; B.S. Rathor, H.C. Mathur, S. Saxena, "Nutritional Anthropometry of 1000 Children Dwelling in the Slum Areas of Jaipur Compared to that of 500 Children of the Elite," *Indian Journal of Pediatrics* 42 (September 1977), 264-76.
11. Chatterjee, G.C., "Nutritional Problems of India," *Science and Culture* 42 (1976), 3.
12. *Ibid.*, p. 3.
13. Aykroyd, W.R., "Conquest of Deficiency Diseases: Protein-Calorie Malnutrition," *Indian Journal of Medical Science* 25 (1971), 415-30.
14. Sukhatme, P.V., "Protein Deficiency in Urban and Rural Areas," *Proceedings of the Nutrition Society 29th Annual Meeting* (London: n.p., May 1970), p. 176.
15. *Ibid.*, p. 179.
16. Rao, T.M.V., *et al.*, "Nutritional Status of Children in Urban Slums Around Delhi," *Indian Journal of Medical Research* (October 1974).
17. Gopalan, C., *et al.*, *Diet Atlas of India*, p. 19.
18. Gopalan, C. and B.S. Narsingha Rao, "Nutritional Constraints on Growth and Development in Current Indian Dietaries," *Indian Journal of Medical Research* 59 (June 1971), 116-17.
19. Husain, S. Sajid, "Nutritional Deficiency Diseases in Badaun and Sahahjahanpur Districts," *The Geographer* 16 (1967), 45-56; Ali Zahoor Khan, "Nutritional Deficiency Disease and Environmental Factors in the Central Ganga-Yamana Doab," *The Geographer* 16 (1969), 57-77.

20. Blyn, George, "Nutritional Adequacy of Punjab and Haryana Cultivator Families," paper presented at the Sixth Annual Wisconsin Conference on South Asia, University of Wisconsin-Madison, 6 November, 1977.
21. Schoefield, Sue and C.M. Lambart, (ed)., *Village Nutrition Studies: An Annotated Bibliography* (Sussex: Institute of Development Studies, University of Sussex, 1975).
22. *Ibid.*, p. 131.
23. Azad, R.N., "Nutrition in the Context of Food Shortage and Rising Population," *Kurukshetra* 23 (February 1975), 11-13.
24. *Ibid.*, p. 13, Grade III is acute form of PCM, whereas Grade II and Grade I are moderate and mild form of PCM, respectively.
25. Gopalan, C. and Raghavan, *Nutritional Atlas*, pp. 104-5.
26. See for example: Bhandari, *et al.*, "Nutritional Anthropometry of Rural School Children of Udaipur District," *Indian Journal of Pediatrics* 39 (January 1972), p. 1-11; Levinson, Morinda: *An Economic Analysis*; Perenia, "Growth of Children in Tamilnadu," pp. 164-76; T.M. V. Rao, "Nutritional Status of Children in Urban Slums Around Delhi,: D.S. Miller and P.R. Payne, "Assessment of Protein Requirements, *Proceedings of Nutrition Society* 28 (1969): 225; D.S. McLaren and P.L. Pell, "Nutrition in the Middle East, in *World Review of Nutrition and Dietetics*, Vol. 12 (New York: Kargar, 1970), pp. 43-127.
27. For empirical findings see: John B. Wyon and E. John, *The Khanna Study: Population Problems in the Rural Punjab* (Cambridge: Harvard University Press, 1971); Ajit Kumar, Y.C. Mathur and Harish Chander, "A Study of the Morbidity Pattern Amongst Pre-School Children in a Rural Area," *Indian Pediatrics*, 9 (1972), 327-31; N.D. Banik, *et al.*, "A Study of Epidemiologic Basis of Malnutrition in Pre-School Children in Slum Areas in Delhi," *Indian Pediatrics* 10 (January, 1973): 25.
28. Schoefield and Lambart, Village Nutrition Studies, pp. 129-130; T.M. Planalp, *Heat Stress and Culture in North India* (Natick, Mass: U.S. Army Research Institute, 1971); S.C. Sharma, "Land Use and Nutrition in the Village Manikpur in the Central Upland of the Lower Yamuna Chambal Doab," *The Geographical Review of India* 34 (1972): 369-385.
29. C. Gopalan, and Nandamuni Naidu, "Nutrition and Fertility," *Lancet* (November 18, 1972), 1077-79; D.M. Heer and D.O. Smith, "Mortality Level, Desired Family Size, and Population Increase," *Demography* 5 (1968): 104-21; K.K. Khanna, "Nutrition and Population," *Indian Pediatrics*; Wyon and Gordon, *Khanna Study.*
30. Chaudhri, M.K., "Nutrition Profile of Calcutta Pre-School Children: Clinical Observations," *Indian Journal of Medical Research* 63 (February 1975), 189-95; Pereria, "Growth Tamilnadu," pp. 164-76; N.R. Bhandari and G.P. Pateel, "Dietary and Feeding Habits of Infants in Various Socio-Economic Groups," *Indian Pediatrics* 10

(April 1973), 233-8; A.S. Chikermane, Socio-Cultural and Economic Aspects of Infant Feeding and Malnutrition," *Indian Pediatrics* 12 (January 1975), 20-21; N.S. Deodhar, "Social and Cultural Factors Conditioning Infant Feeding" *Indian Journal of Medical Science* 21 (November 1967), 770-72: Chakravarti, "Regional Preference for Food."

31. Chakravarti, "Regional Preferences in India."
32. Ghai, O.P., Feeding Habits in Relation to Diarrhea and Malnutrition," *Indian Pediatrics* 12 (1975), 72.
33. Generally, there is a folk-belief that certain foods, such as eggplant, are heat producing and should not be consumed in summer. Likewise, certain foods, such as yogurt, are avoided during winter due to their cold-producing effect on the physiological system; see Table 6.8.
34. Gopalan, C., *et al., Diet Atlas of India*, p. 19.
35. Levinson, "Morinda: An Economic Analysis of Malnutrition."
36. A detailed discussion on different aspects of maternal and child nutrition planning in India, theoretical as well as applied, is initiated in Indian Council of Medical Research, *Alternative Approaches to Health Care.*
37. Leonard Joy, "Food and Nutrition Planning," *Journal of Agricultural Economics* 34 (January, 1973), 184.
38. Government of India, *Fourth Five Year Plan* (New Delhi: Government of India Publications, 1973), p. 244.
39. Berg, Alan, *The Nutrition Factor: Its Role in National Development* (Washington, D.C.: The Brookings Institution, 1973), pp. 188-92.

# 3

# Conceptualization of the Malnutrition Problem

## A GEO-ECOLOGICAL PERSPECTIVE

MALNUTRITION is a complex problem to solve. The complexity lies in its multidimensional underpinning of etiological and ecological factors. If we want to know why a balanced diet is not available or consumed by a population in a particular socio-economic or biological group or in an area (ecological zone), an understanding of the mutual relationship of several factors, as mentioned in Fig. 3.1, is essential. Although most of the earlier studies recognize the contribution of such factors in influencing nutritional status, a holistic treatment (with ecosystem perspective) has been attempted by few scholars. A theoretical approach of this nature for surveillance of nutritional needs in a community is well illustrated in a technical report of WHO.[1] In analyzing the problem from a complete systems perspective, Tamilnadu's study is the only study known to the author.[2]

The ecological and systems[3] (Ecosystem) perspectives, because of their holistic and integrative nature, appear to be more appealing for nutrition analysis than the piecemeal approaches. Nutrition status is not explainable by isolated domains; rather, an interrelation of several subsystems (domains) is apparent (Fig. 3.1). A theoretical basis for such interactions and interrelations is presented in the following discussion to elucidate the possible outcomes in the statistical analysis as presented in Chapter 6. Since the child's nutrition status in the

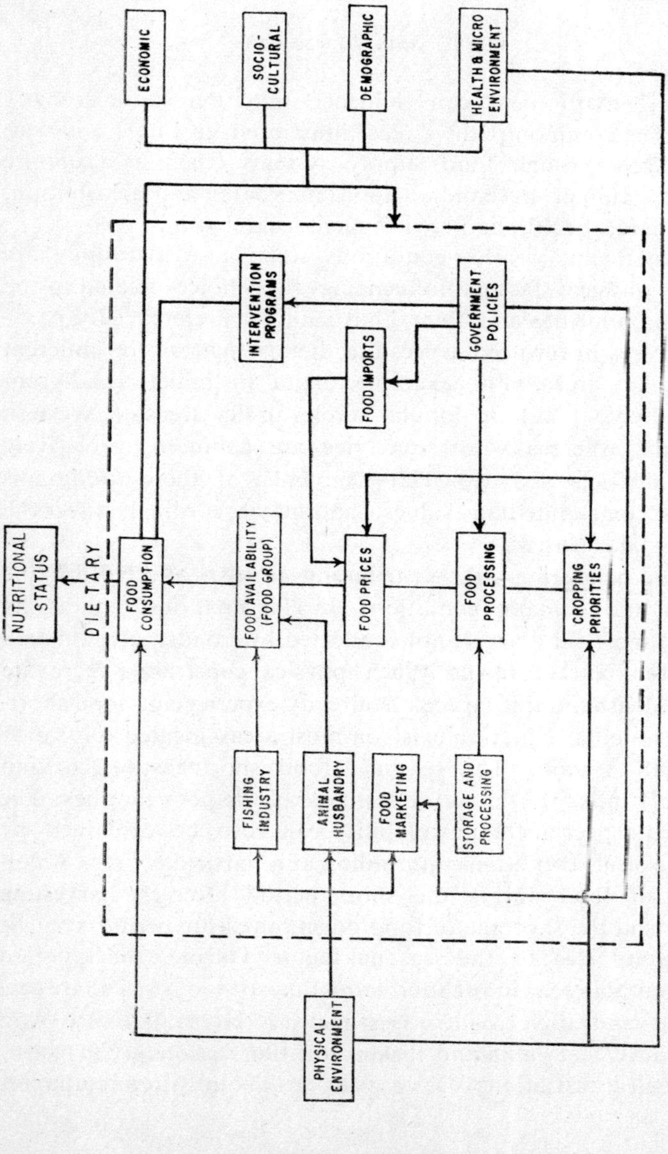


FIG. 3.1 : *Intercorrelations of Factors Influencing Nutritional Status*

short run is influenced by the family life style and health related factors, only selected domains (such as economic, socio-cultural, demographic, health, physical environment) will be discussed which have direct bearing on the dietary pattern of the children.[4]

## PHYSICAL ENVIRONMENT

Physical environment can influence nutrition status in many ways. The common pathway as illustrated in Fig. 3.1 is conceptualized through food supply systems (such as cropping priority, animal husbandry, food marketing and distribution, and fishing), health, and environmental sanitation.

Climatic and weather conditions, soils, and hydrology are clearly physical factors influencing the choices related to the cropping priorities and animal husbandry. Preference for particular crops, in turn, influences the dietary pattern in different geographic areas. For example, bajra (a millet), and gram (kind of chickpeas) are popular staples in dry areas of Western Haryana, whereas wheat and rice are common in relatively humid districts of North Haryana. Each of these foodgrains has different nutrition values, and may accordingly affect the nutritional status.

Food marketing and distribution is also affected by the terrain and climatic conditions. In Haryana, during the rainy season, most rural areas, not connected by roads, are isolated from the market towns. Such physical constraints aggravate the food situation, if an area is already experiencing food shortages. A similar situation exists in most areas located in sandy and hilly terrain. The seasonal food shortages of this kind evidently influence the nutrient intake of the poor families. The seasonal aspect of food availability can also be explained by the physical conditions prevailing at a particular time. Availability of food during the short period after the harvesting season and the shortage of food during the lean period can be understood due to the seasonal factor. During a slack period (unfavourable season for food crops) most food stocks are exhausted and high food prices restrict the availability. At a global level, Newman and Pickett mention seasonality in terms of climatic variations. They warn us about the consequences of such variability in food supplies resulting in famines and large food deficits in the dry and variable climate areas.[5]

Physical environments also promote certain vectored diseases and hence influence the morbidity-nutritional status pattern of an area. For example, swamps and dense vegetation in heavy rainfall or irrigated areas promote the origin and transmission of several vectored diseases such as malaria and schistosomiasis. The onslaught of such periodic infections results in low food intake and hence debilitates the child. Within deficiency diseases, the incidence of endemic goiter in the mountainous and sub-mountain regions is due to the deficiency of iodine in the water and soil. The food crops grown are, therefore, deficient in this nutrient and precipitate endemic goiter. The influence of several "geographical" factors in causing deficiency diseases has been very well explained by Patwardhan and May,[6] and need not be discussed here.

The climatic rhythms also influence the seasonality of diseases. According to Planalp, most infectious diseases in North India have their highest incidence during the dry seasons. The seasonality effect is also felt in the accessibility of the urban and rural health facilities. During the rainy season, people may not be able to reach them conveniently due to poor transportation links. The morbidity rate is apparently exacerbated as a result of poor accessibility.

From the above discussion it is apparent that physical environment is a kind of control subsystem, and the variation in its components affects its relationship with other subsystems (such as food and health) and consequently the nutrition system. The impact of this domain in the present study will be analyzed in a more descriptive manner. The concern is to analyze how physical conditions in general have influenced the food availability, and general health conditions of the studied children in the sampled villages.

## INCOME DOMAIN

Among the determinants of malnutrition, no other factor seems to affect the nutritional status of the children as much as family income. Due to the skewed distribution of income in the LDC's, only a small portion of the population has enough purchasing

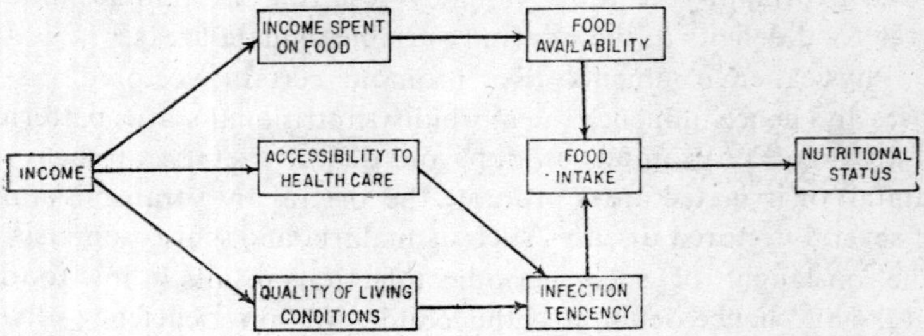


FIG. 3.2 : *Influence of income on the Nutritional Status*

power to include expensive nutritious foods, primarily of animal origin, in their food budgets. Several food consumption and anthropometric studies done in India (see Chapter 2) clearly indicate nutritional status variation along the income spectrum. How a family's purchasing power (including income, commodity prices, and other demands on a family budget) influences the nutritional status is illustrated in Fig. 3.2.

**Relation of Income with Food Consumption**

Three universal trends are noticed in food consumption with the increase in income:

(*i*) Increase in amount of food (mostly carbohydrates) with increase in income and the relationship is true up to a limit beyond which the relationship is not strong,

(*ii*) Decrease in calories supplied by the carbohydrate rich staples (cereals mainly), and increased use of expensive nutritious foods of animal and vegetal origin, and

(*iii*) Shift towards variety and more highly processed foods.[8]

Several studies at global,[9] national, regional, or local levels indicate a similar relationship of higher caloric consumption with increasing income. With reference to India, the Indian Council of Medical Research in nationwide surveys has clearly revealed protein and caloric consumption contrasts in urban and rural situations and across high and low income group children. Pre-school children belonging to high income families of urban areas are reported to be about 45 per cent higher in caloric consumption as compared to their counterparts in low income families of rural areas. Such shortages are even true, although of lesser magnitudes, when compared with recommended allowances. Protein variations are not significant between young children of different income groups; however, the gap widens with higher age-groups. By all standards, the relationship between quantity of food and income is clear.

Furthermore, the diet composition also changes substantially with increasing income. The cereal, tuber- or root-based caloric diets are usually observed to be supplemented with more nutritious foods of animal or vegetal origin. Foods such as meat, poultry, legumes, milk, ghee (clarified butter), vegetables, and fruits add variety and quality to the monotonous carbohydrate-rich diets. At the national level, such trends in the diet pattern are stated to be a function of economic development. Three broad generalizations are evident in the diet composition with change in national incomes:

(*i*) Protein supplies change from largely plant to animal origin,

(*ii*) Caloric supplies change primarily from starch-rich foods to fat-rich foods and refined sugar. Saturated and unsaturated fats thus become the principal source of concentrated energy, and

(*iii*) Cereal content of the diet is inversely proportional to the income.

In economic terms, the changes in diet pattern are also reflected by the income elasticity of demand for various food products. Based on a FAO food survey, Call and Levinson state that in Asia and the Far East (excluding Japan) the elasticities of vegetables, meat, and eggs are estimated at 0.9, .5 and 2.0 respectively, while the elasticity for cereal is 0.5.[10] The authors further contend that these elasticities decrease, and tend to be higher in rural than in urban areas. Such demand for more expensive foods may not always be translated exactly into nutritional increments. There is an interesting qualitative change in the food behavior of people as income increases. For example, people may shift from less expensive coarse grains such as jowar (sorgum) and bajra (millets) to expensive food-grains such as wheat flour and polished rice.[11] A comprehensive survey in Maharashtra state revealed that the percentage of families eating wheat increased from 21 per cent in the rural areas (low income), which is almost in reverse proportion to the numbers eating jowar. The literature abounds with examples of shifts from brown bread to white bread, brown rice to polished rice, margerine to butter, peanuts to almonds and jaggery to refined sugar.

Similar negative effects of income are also observed in poor infant feeding practices. A significant decline in breast-feeding and increasing popularity of bottle-feeding has been noticed, particularly among mothers belonging to rich families, and those living in the urban areas.[12] In a study of Indian women, over 80 per cent of the highest socio-economic groups did not breast-feed their infants for more than six months, while among the lowest socio-economic classes such a practice was practically unknown.[13] The nutritional outcomes of bottle-feeding are found damaging in the poor countries. Unsanitary preparation of the formula with the contaminated water and general unhygienic conditions often lead to higher incidences of diarrhea or other debilitating illness, rather than improving the nutritional status.

In brief, we can say that for the population as a whole, increases in income may be automatically translated into adequate and quality food, which, in turn, leads to improved nutritional status. The negative effects of income may be evident, mainly in very high income families, where nutritional status may not rise in accordance with increase in income.

## Relation of Income in Maintaining Health Status

The effect of income on health can be illustrated through quality of living conditions and accessibility to the health care facilities. Due to less expendable income, the quality of living conditions is usually substandard in most low income families. Such poor living conditions are typically reflected in high rooming density, poor house maintenance, absence of garbage disposal and collecting facilities, unsanitary environment, and unhygienic habits. Consequently, the probability of contracting communicable and parasitic diseases is obviously higher in the low income children.

Succinctly stated, the multifaceted relationship of income to several surrogates of food and health makes it a major determinant of nutritional status. A careful analysis of this domain is, therefore, needed for an indepth understanding of the malnutrition problem.

## SOCIO-CULTURAL DOMAIN

### Social Factors

The social impact on the N.S. is illustrated here principally through the work status of the mother. Work status of the mother affects the N.S. of a child in two ways. The working mothers cannot provide the quality care needed by the child during his early development. At this time, the fulfilment of physiological, emotional, and nutritional needs is crucial for the healthy development of the child. If adequate child care facilities are not available in a community, the health status of children belonging to working mothers is expected to be lower than that of those belonging to non-working mothers. Since child care facilities are inadequate in rural Haryana, the inverse relationship of N.S. with working mothers is expected in the present study.

Furthermore, female participation in labor force in rural Haryana generally varies with caste structure. This is particularly high among Hindu Jat, Ahir, Gujjar, and scheduled caste families. Economic necessity, as is true for most scheduled castes, or social norms to help the husbands, as common in Hindu Jats, Ahirs, and Gujjars, generally leads to female participation in most farming operations except plowing. Due to this typical association of caste and female participation in the work-force, the N.S. of the mentioned castes' children is expected to be low.

### Cultural Factors

Cultural factors, such as religion and caste, not only have bearing on what people prefer to eat but also on what they grow (cropping pattern) and distribute in the economic system. There-is abundant literature indicating that the cultural impact on food intake of the adults or children is guided by societal norms.[14] Cultural relativism generally dictates the preferences and prejudices for variety of animal or vegetal origin foods. Feeding and weaning practices, methods of preparation, distribution system within the family, and preservation methods are noticed to be greatly influenced by socio-cultural standards.

In the Indian context, such cultural influences on the food intake can be understood through caste and religious differences.[15] Caste rules often monitor the kinds of food a man may eat or abstain from. The people of higher caste (particularly Brahmins) abstain from eating flesh foods, whereas the lowest castes (the so-called untouchables) have no such prescription, although both groups may belong to the Hindu religion. Caste differences are also observed in growing crops and raising animals. The Sikhs, for example, do not grow eggplant, and the Hindus do not raise chickens. Likewise, feeding and weaning practices also vary across castes. Prolonged breast-feeding is common among the cultivating castes (particularly Jats), whereas early weaning is usual among the rich business castes (Bania) of Haryana. The nutritional differences due to such cultural variations in the food habits are, therefore, obvious, and may be reflected in the varying nutritional standard of different castes' children.

Religion is another major cultural element which leads to faulty food habits, and thus to nutritional disorders. Some nutritious foods in India are not consumed strictly due to religious aphorism. The non-vegetarian maxim of food among most staunch Hindus, Jains and Budhists prohibits them from eating flesh foods due to the religious code of ahimsa (a moral code of non-violence and respect for every form of life). On the other hand, the Sikhs, Muslims, and many lower caste Hindus attach little taboo to eating meat or poultry. Contrary to the general belief that most Indians (Hindus) are vegetarians, the Indian Institute of Nutrition in a national sample survey has observed that more than 60 per cent of the urban population and about 75 per cent of the rural population listed themselves as non-vegetarians.[16] The study further contends that most subjects of low income are vegetarians because of economic necessity. Since no data on the amount or frequency of non-vegetarian foods are given, the data need to be interpreted with caution. The findings of this nature exhort that cultural norms sometimes get entrenched in a society due to economic reality rather than of religiosity. In nutrition studies such concerns need to be explored more carefully such that the real needs of the community can be identified based on their food habits, and other related factors.

## DEMOGRAPHIC DOMAIN

Until recently, the relationship of malnutrition with domains such as population was either less emphasized or dismissed on the basis of obscurity. Population control programs had rarely stressed the complementarity of family size and the health status of the young children. The solutions to both problems have usually been pursued independent of each other. More recently, however, the nutrition experts are trying to impress that integrated solutions to both problems can be achieved if the relationship between the two is made clear. The theoretical basis and empirical evidence suggest that the malnutrition problem is generally aggravated in large families, and where the children are closely spaced.[17] Both size and spacing variables influence the availability of food and the morbidity rate, which in turn, affect the nutritional status of the child. The apparent relationship between health of the children (N.S.) and some demographic variables is illustrated in Fig. 3.3.

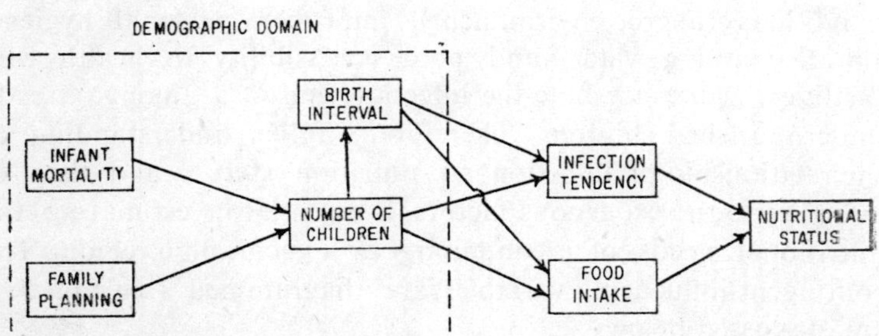


FIG. 3.3 : *Influence of Demographic Variables on the Nutritional Status*

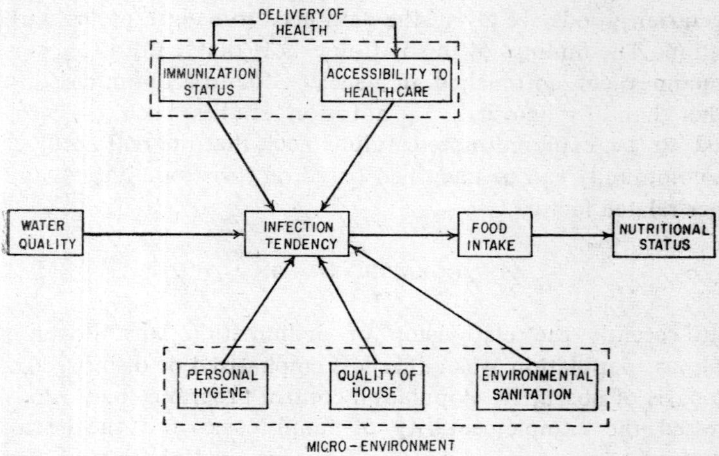


FIG. 3.4 : *Possible Causes of Infection and Its Relation with Nutritional Status*

THE HEALTH DOMAIN

The close synergistic relationship of pediatric malnutrition and infection in the less developed countries has been well documented by Scrimshaw and others.[18] These scholars postulate that even if the right foods are available to the child, they may not have their full impact upon growth unless the infections are corrected. The exogenous factors, such as unhygienic living conditions (micro environment), improper personal hygiene, unsafe drinking water, and poor accessibility to health care facilities, can exacerbate the infection episodes among already undernourished children. Therefore, a fuller understanding of the relationship of infection to nutrition status, and then of infection to the exogenous factors, is essential in estimating the nutritional needs of a community or a geographic region. The contingent influencing variables are diagrammed (see Fig. 3.4) and discussed below:

**Micro-Environment**

The micro-environment in the present context is referred to as the matrix of the most immediate physical-social surroundings of the child and generally reflects the quality of living conditions. Its relationship with infectious diseases can be best understood by the medical geography concept of agent/host/environment relationship.[19] According to May, the geographical factors—"geogens"—(such as overcrowding, damp air, and unsanitary conditions) have a provisional relationship with disease causing agents—pathogens—(such as viruses, bacteria, fungi) or vectors (such as arthropods). The pathogens can be transmitted directly (as in case of influenza) or indirectly through vector (as in case of malaria) into the susceptible host (the undernourished child here) under the typical environmental conditions. In order to break this disease-producing cycle, the child's environment seems the most intervenable element. Therefore, a detailed understanding of the quality of living conditions is desirable to mitigate the malnutrition/infection synergism. The quality of living conditions can be evaluated and classified into good, moderate, and poor on the subjective examination of the following elements:

(*i*) Location and building material of the house,
(*ii*) Air circulation and sunlight conditions in the living quarters,
(*iii*) Density of living rooms,
(*iv*) Location of animal quarters in relation to family's living space, and
(*v*) Sanitary disposal and personal hygiene.

Rural conditions in India, and in Haryana in particular, are generally marked by compact settlements to the extent that most dwellings have three common walls with their neighbours. The compactness facilitates dissemination of communicable diseases under strong caste and neighborly affinity. As regards quality of construction and building material, most houses are usually built of adobe blocks with mud plaster and no stone foundation. Dirt floors and walls allow young children to come in contact with several disease agents such as parasites and enteropathogenic bacteria. During the rainy and stormy weather conditions, the drafty and leaky dwellings often enhance the prevalence of respiratory infections (such as the common cold).

The compact layout further diminishes the prospect of air circulation and sunshine in most dwellings. The hot and humid conditions are ideal for the multiplication of pathogens and several vectors, which in turn help in transmitting infectious diseases.

The juxtaposition of houses and cattle sheds, often in single compound, is a common sight in Haryana villages. This unhealthy practice of keeping draft animals in close proximity to human beings is partly resorted to as a safeguard from cattle stealing and shortage of covered space during the winters. Its impact on the health of the children and adults can be notable as a result of unsanitary conditions produced by the animal urine and dung which may carry pathogens. Besides, the unhygienic practice of making dungcakes and piling them into heaps is common around houses located at the edge of the village. The visible effect of such practices in causing infections is beyond the scope of this study, albeit their contribution in producing unsanitary and unhygienic conditions cannot be eluded.

Furthermore, safe sanitary disposal facilities are almost non-existent in Haryana villages. The garbage and trash are usually disposed of either in a fixed corner of the house or thrown out in the street with no collection facility. In absence of any flush or basket toilets, the nearby fields and in some instances streets are used as open latrines by the young children. Besides, in the absence of storm water drainage and sewer facilities, the stagnant pools of water invariably become reservoirs of defecated matter and other human wastes. The young children already suffering from minor ailments or nutritional deficiencies may thus become potential hosts to several water-borne diseases (such as bacillary dysentery, hookworm, cholera, hepatitis, typhoid). The open drains often flowing through the middle of the streets can be the potential source of disease-carrying vectors such as house flies and mosquitoes.

Last, but not least, most families in rural areas are generally little conscious of personal hygiene. Use of common towels and drinking cups, carelessness about handkerchiefs, imperfectly washed dishes and eating utensils, and hands soiled with nasal secretion are familiar practices. Diffusion of some infectious diseases could possibly be related to such unhygienic habits.

**Availability of Quality Water**

It is difficult to know how many people do not have access to a supply of water suitable for drinking. One estimate made by WHO in the early 1970s concluded on the basis of a questionnaire that roughly 72 per cent of the total population in a number of poor nations did not have access to community water supply within a reasonable distance.[20]

By far, the largest number of people with poor access live in the rural areas. The nutritional implications of the inaccessibility to safe drinking water are obvious, since several debilitating diseases in the developing countries are reportedly due to the use of unhealthy and polluted water obtained from open wells, tanks, and ponds. The list of such diseases is long; however, the most debilitating diseases affecting young children include infectious hepatitis, cholera, typhoid, bacillary dysentery, and enterovirus diarrheas.

Although a precise relationship of infections to polluted water is not attempted in this study, the accessibility to safe drinking water may reveal the potential hazard of infections present in different communities and geographic areas. A higher incidence of water-borne infections is expected in the low income groups, untouchables and other lower castes, and in those areas where the possibility of tapping shallow sub-surface water sources is meagre.

**Accessibility to Health Care System**

The problem of high morbidity in the rural areas is further exacerbated by the poor delivery of medical services. Skewed distribution of the trained medical manpower and modern health facilities to the urban areas—especially to the district headquarters, provincial capitals, and metropolitan areas—makes the health services inaccessible and unavailable to most of the rural populace. Indirect factors of transport cost, time cost and behavioral preferences for the traditional medical system also inhibit the adequate use of available facilities. The following examples from India and other developing countries illustrate the inadequacy of the curative aspect of health care in improving or maintaining the health standards in the rural situations.

As regards medical manpower, the per capita availability of qualified medical doctors is not only far below the expected

TABLE 3.1: **Population Per Medical Doctor in Urban and Rural Areas in Selected Countries**

| Country | Year | Population/Medical Doctor | | |
|---|---|---|---|---|
| | | Nationwide | Urban | Rural |
| Pakistan | 1970 | 7,400 | 3,700 | 24,200 |
| Kenya | 1969 | 12,140 | 800 | 50,000 |
| Philippines | 1971 | 3,900 | 1,500 | 10,000 |
| Honduras | 1968 | 3,860 | 1,190 | 7,140 |
| Columbia | 1970 | 2,160 | 1,000 | 6,400 |
| Iran | 1967-70 | 3,752 | 2,275 | 10,000 |
| Panama | 1969 | 1,790 | 930 | 3,000 |

*Source*: World Bank, *Health*: Sector Policy Paper, March 1975, p. 80.

norms, but also highly concentrated in the urban areas. Table 3.1 illustrates the quantitative gap of the latter type in a few selected countries.

Even with the expanding health facilities, the informal health system, mainly the folk practitioners, seems to provide the bulk of health needs of the rural communities. Recent health need studies on India indicate that less than 20 per cent of the rural sick population consult qualified doctors of the Western Medicine System, around 65 per cent go to the indigenous type practitioners, and the rest either do not consult or practice self treatment.[21] Although better data on this aspect are needed, the general trend is not significantly different.[22] Notwithstanding the contribution of traditional practitioners in providing inexpensive and easily accessible health care, their professional effectiveness in scientific terms is usually argued and debated by the modern health system. The nutrition aspect is of particular concern at this point. For example, most Indian physicians of the indigenous system often restrict or avoid the use of food products such as yogurt, cold beverages, citrus fruits, and most fruit juices, during the common cold or cough episodes. Cereals, legumes, meat and eggs are also restricted foods during most common fevers. Restrictions of this nature naturally have nutritional implications.

Not only the medical doctors but the modern health facilities too are oriented to an urban population. In spite of the increasing government efforts to expand health facilities in rural

TABLE 3.2: **Health Center Outreach (Including Sub Centers)**

| | |
|---|---|
| Population never using PHC services | 77.0 per cent |
| Proportion of morbidities attended | 10.4 per cent |
| Patients beyond two miles | 14.5 per cent |
| Female patients beyond two miles | 8.4 per cent |
| Proportion of infants covered by MCH Programs | 20.0 per cent |
| Visits per infant (Yearly) | 1.2 per cent |
| Coverage of infants beyond two miles | 9.0 per cent |
| Coverage of antenatal cases beyond two miles | 7.3 per cent |
| Deliveries beyond two miles | 8.0 per cent |
| Proportion of female patients in O.P.D. | 33.7 per cent |

*Source*: Indian Council of Medical Research and Indian Council of Social Research, *Alternate Approaches to Health Care* (New Delhi: Indian Council of Medical Research, c. 1977).

areas, the outreach of such facilities is limited to a small population within a two or three mile radius of their location. The magnitude of the quantitative gap between health needs of rural population and the actual outreach of the existing services, in the case of one rural block of India, is illustrated by Table 3.2.

The above discussion evidently indicates that neither the preventive nor the curative aspects of health care in rural India are adequate enough to contain the infectious diseases common among the young children. In Haryana, where the environmental sanitation conditions and delivery of health systems are not satisfactory, the infectious episodes are likely to be one of the principal contributing factors of malnutrition.

## DIETARY DOMAIN

Among the family-community ecology factors discussed so far, there can be no better indicator of the nutritional status than the availability of food to the individual child. Due to its direct bearing on the metabolism, diet is of particular importance in regulating the nutritional conditions in young children.

Notwithstanding the great significance of this domain in assessing directly the nutritional adequacies or inadequacies, the real problem exists in using the right kind of dietary indicators to predict the nutritional status. Realizing this kind of problem,

Sanjur and Romero suggest five alternative approaches—dietary complexity, food diversity, food quantity, proteic food score, and nutritional assessment—to predict the nutritional status of young children from the dietary data.[23] Use of a particular method of course depends on the purpose, feasibility and objectives of the study. The food diversity method is preferred here as the precise recording and weighing of food (based on the 24-hour recall method) is difficult in the rural conditions. This becomes even more difficult when breast-feeding is a common practice and mothers do not follow a schedule in feeding children. Furthermore, factors of cost and time constitute barriers to the utilization of food weighing techniques. Thus, the food diversity level offers a meaningful alternative to dietary assessment.

Food diversity is defined here as a function of a single or a combination of food groups available to a child during a l-day period. Four types of food groups are thought to be possible in the diet patterns of rural young children:

(*i*) Protein dominant food group (for very young children),
(*ii*) Carbohydrate rich food group,
(*iii*) Mixed food group (combination of group I and group II), and
(*iv*) Balanced food group (group III and inclusion of vegetables, fruits, and lipids).

In the present study, nutritional status of a child is supposed to vary with the kind of food group ingested. The healthier children are expected in group III and group IV, as they contain a variety of foods with essential nutrients. On the other hand, protein dominant (mainly mother's milk) and carbohydrate rich (primarily cereals) food groups are hypothesized to contain less healthy children due to either absence or insufficiency of many protective food elements available in the former food groups. The problem may be less severe in protein group if the child is very young and depends on breast-feeding.

Several reasons can be accountable for inclusion of one food group and exclusion of others in the family's diet. Many of such factors have already been mentioned in the earlier literature review and conceptualization. In short, income, size of the family, age of the child, health conditions, food habits of the family, and physical conditions conducive to the growth of food crops usually affect the availability of a particular food group. Additionally, the secondary factors of urbanization and Green Revolution cannot be ignored in the availability of certain foods to the rural populace. For example, the growing demand for vegetables, fruits, and milk in the urban areas has led to almost an exclusion of such foods in the diet pattern of the rural poor. Similarly, the Green Revolution impact is felt from the declining acreage and production of leguminous crops, whereas the foodgrains and other commercial crops are gaining priority due to their high yielding varieties. Such a trend is typically true in most green revolution states, such as Haryana. Evidently, both direct and indirect factors are responsible in making a particular food group available to a child. Influences of this nature need to be examined in explaining the relationship of food group to the nutritional status.

**Summary**

The conceptualization outlined above clearly demonstrates that malnutrition is a complex problem because of its underpinnings in several domains. The complexity is further compounded by the interrelated nature of several causative determinants or indicators of malnutrition. Some determinants seem to have direct bearing while the others are tangential to the problem. In order to precisely estimate the causes of malnutrition (PCM in this study) we need to zero in on those indicators which are directly related to the problem and can be subjected to statistical analysis and later used for planned measures. Furthermore, for statistical analysis, few independent variables can be more meaningful in explaining the causality of malnutrition than several interrelated variables that may have only indirect bearing to the nutritional status. With this view in mind, the hypothesized relationship of the mentioned domains will be ascertained with the possible determinants as identified in Table 3.3. The supporting variables in the Table are those indicators that help in explaining the determinants and will not be subjected to statistical analysis for prediction or causal relationship with the nutritional status.

TABLE 3.3: **Possible Determinants and Associated Variables of Malnutrition**

| Domain | Determinant | Supporting Variables |
|---|---|---|
| Health and Micro-Environment | Infection Tendency | Immunization, Source of Drinking Water, Personal Hygiene, Density per Room |
| | Quality of Living Conditions | Sanitary Conditions, Rubbish Disposal, Location of Animal Rooms, Air Circulation |
| Dietary | Food Groups of the child | Age of the Child, Income of Family, Food Habits |
| Demographic | Number of Children Birth Interval | Family Planning, Education of Mother, Feeding Practices (for Birth Interval) |
| Economic | Annual Income | Occupation |
| Socio-cultural | Work status of Mother, Occupation, Caste structure | |

In brief, our effort here is to isolate the principal correlates responsible for the causation of malnutrition in a community or a geographic area. Later, the statistical analysis will help us bring out their relative contribution to explain the nutritional status variation in the studied population. The methods used for this purpose are given in Chapter 4.

## REFERENCES

1. World Health Organization, *Methodology of Nutritional Surveillance*, Technical Report Series 593 (Geneva: World Health Organization: 1976).
2. Sol Chafkin, "An Operations Oriented Study of Nutrition as an Integrated System of Tamilnadu" (report prepared for Food and Nutrition Division, U.S. Agency for International Development/New Delhi, February 11, 1970).

3. For a theoretical understanding of the systems approach, a cogent account is given by F. Kenneth Berrien, *Ganeral and Social Systems* (New Jersey: Rutgers University Press, 1968; Von Bertaslanfey, General Systems Theory (New York: George Bra-Zillar, 1968); and Ervin Laszlo, *Introduction to Systems Philosophy* (New York: Harper and Row Publishers, 1972). For systems approach in nutrition, see Alan Berg and Robert Muscat, "Nutrition Program Planning: An Approach" in *Nutrition, National Development and Planning*, (ed). Alan Berg, Nevin S. Scrimshaw and David L. Call (Cambridge, Mass: The MIT Press), pp. 247-74; S.R. Simm, *et al., A Systems Approach to the World Protein Problem.* Report prepared by the Battelle Memorial Institute for the United Nations Protein Advisory Group, May 6, 1970. The concept of ecosystem as applied in geography to understand the environmental and host of socio-economic-cultural interactions is lucidly given by Stoddart, "Geography and Ecological Approach," and R.J. Chorley "Geography As Human Ecology" in *Directions in Geography*, ed. Richard T. Chorley (London: Methuen & Company 1973), pp. 155-70.
4. For clarity sake it may be added that nutrition problem as a whole is treated as a mega-system. The mega-system is composed of several domains which directly or indirectly influence the N.S. Each domain is further influenced by or related to several determinants or supporting variables. The following discussion on each domain is an attempt to understand the interrelationships of the components and sub-components of the malnutrition mega-system.
5. Newman, E. James and Robert C. Pickett, "World climates and Food Supply Variations," *Science* 186 (December 6, 1974), 877-81.
6. Patwardhan, "Geographic Distribution of Malnutrition,"; May, *The Ecology of Human Diseases.*
7. Planalp, *Heat Stress in North India.*
8. Call, David L. and F. James Levinson, "A Systematic Approach to Nutrition Intervention Programs," in *Nutritional National Development*, ed. Berg *et al.*, pp. 167-69.
9. Knight, C. Gregary and R. Paul Wilcox, *Triumph or Triage: The World Food Problem in Geographical Perspective*, AAG Resource Paper 75-3 (Washington, D.C.: Association of American Geographers, 1976).
10. Call and Levinson, "A Systems Approach to Nutrition," p. 168.
11. It may be mentioned that both jowar and bajra are higher in protein, fat, mineral, and vitamins content than rice. Wheat is not significantly different in nutrients but almost twice in price of the coarse grains.
12. Among several causes leading to bottle-feeding the most important include: bottle as a status symbol, changing social attitudes toward sexual attractiveness, convenience, aggressive sales promotion tactics, and increasing women participating in the work-force.

13. Gopalan, C., "Studies on Lactation in Poor Indian Communities," *Journal of Tropical Pediatrics* (December 1958), 92.
14. For a variety of studies see C.S. Wilson, *Food Habits: A Selected Annotated Bibliography*, Journal of Nutrition Education, 5 (Supplement 1973).
15. See in particular Rajmal P. Devdas, "Social and Cultural Factors Influencing Mulnutrition" *Journal of Home Economics*, 62 (March 1973), 164-71; A.K. Chakravarti, "Regional Preferences for Food in India"; R.K. Golikere, *Vegetarianism vs. Non-Vegetarianism* (Bombay: Popular Books, 1960); P. Roy, "The Sacred Cow in India," *Rural Sociology* 20 (1955), 8-15; A.S. Chikermane, "Social-Cultural and Economic Aspects of Infants Feeding and Malnutrition," *Indian Pediatrics* 12 (1975), 20-21.
16. Gopalan, C. *et al.*, *Diet Atlas of India*, pp. 48-49.
17. Austin, James E. and F. James Levinson, "Population and Nutrition: A Case for Integration," *Milbank Memoral Fund Quarterly* 52 (1974), 169-84, Agit Kumar *et al.*, "A Study of the Morbidity in Pre-School Children of Rural Hyderabad in Relation to Family Size and Birth Interval," *Indian Pediatrics* 21 (1976), 123-26.
18. Scrimshaw, Nevin, S. Carl E. Taylor, and John E. Gordon, *Interaction of Nutrition and Infection* (Geneva: World Health Organization, 1968); N.S. Scrimshaw, "Synergism of Malnutrition and Infection: Evidence from Field Studies in Guatemala," *Journal of American Medical Association,* 212 (1970); 1685-92.
19. For a detailed discussion on this topic see Jacques M. May, "Medical Geography: Its Methods and Objectives," *Geographical Review* 40 (1950), 9-41.
20. WHO, *World Health Statistics Report*, Vol. 26, No. 11, 1973, Sec. II, p. 727.
21. John Hopkins University, *Functional Analysis of Health Needs and Services,* Mimeographed (Baltimore: Department of International Health, 1970).
22. For comparison see S. Andrews, "*Feasibility of Involving Indigenous Medical Practitioner for Family Planning Services Delivery in Kerala, India,*" Ph. D. Dissertation, John Hopkins University, 1973.
23. Sanjur, D. and E. Romero, "Conceptual Levels of Dietary Indicators as Predictors of Nutritional Status," *Nutrition* 2 (1975), 214-22.

# 4

# Research Design and Methodology

THIS chapter is designed to illustrate the activities to accomplish the objectives outlined in Chapter 1. The chapter is divided into three sections. The first section deals with the general problems of data availability in the health area. The second pertains to the selection of data points and the households for generating nutrition data on the pre-school children. The third section addresses methodological issues in analyzing the determinants of malnutrition for the survey data and spatial variables.

## WHY USE SURVEY RESEARCH?

The use of survey research is preferred in this study since published anthropometric data and family ecology data in determining the prevalence and causes of malnutrition are generally not available at the micro level. Furthermore, insights into the causes of human malnutrition are reinforced only by field observation. Some of the crucial determinants of malnutrition, such as quality of life conditions—environmental sanitation, personal hygiene, crowding—related to several infectious diseases cannot be estimated without a field investigation. Similarly, the influence of other critical determinants such as the food group available to the child cannot be precisely determined unless we know the food behavior of the family related to feeding practices, weaning foods and food preferences and avoidances. A wide array of information embedded in the family life style or local ecology is, therefore, essential before determining the precise causes of

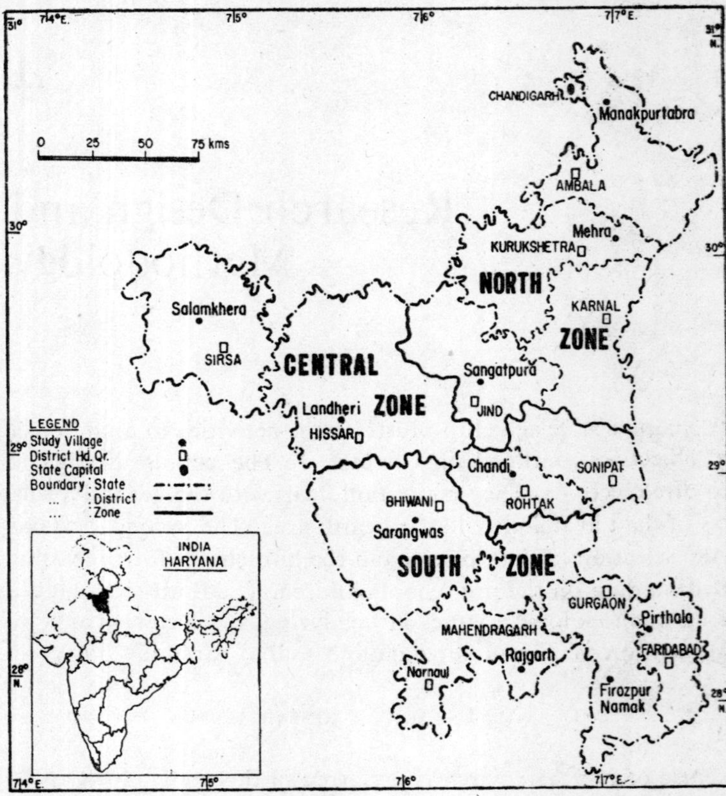


FIG. 4.1 : *Location of Study Zones and Villages of Haryana*

malnutrition. Published data of this nature are hardly available at the village level. Nutrition surveys in Haryana have been primarily of clinical or anthropometric nature, and their emphasis has remained on the prevalence of malnutrition rather than its causes. Realizing the need for field study, the following steps were initiated in generating the nutritional status and family ecology related data.

The selection of data points and other data units (the respondents) was made from the derived ecological zones of the study area (see Fig. 4.1). These zones served two general purposes. First, the derived zones represent a certain degree of regional homogeneity (in terms of climate, soil, agricultural practices, and caste structure), and thus become the first step toward scientific selection of data points (villages). Second, spatial comparisons of a general nature, and knowledge about the study area can be attempted through such a regional division scheme. It may be mentioned, however, that by proposing the regional scheme, it is not assumed that this is necessarily a gradient in the degree of malnutrition. What is assumed is that different factors may be operative in these regions bearing upon the nutritional status.

**Regional Division Scheme**

The state of Haryana, located in the western part of the Indo-Gangetic Plain of India, is the general study area. Geography of this state reveals several regional variations in its physical (see Fig. 4.2), economic, and cultural landscape. These variations can be noticed in relief and landform types, climate, economic activities, social habits, folklore, and even dialects. Such regional diversities can be scanned from the multidisciplinary works of Chib, Lal, Prakash, Singh and Schwartzberg.[1] Singh has mentioned an extraordinary spatial variation in relief and land form types (see Fig. 4.2), climate and edaphic conditions, ground water resources, and irrigation facilities. Cultural diversity as reflected in caste structure and dialects is well documented by Prakash. Bhalla, based on his intensive study of 2,000 households, has observed significant regional diversities in household income, food consumption, savings, and family size for different categories of cultivators and landless laborers of Haryana.[2]

The state has been divided into three zones on the basis of a combination of four major criteria: (*i*) per cent of area irrigated, (*ii*) major soil types, (*iii*) household income, and (*iv*) geographical continuity.[3] In addition, while delineating these zones, major landforms, climatic and edaphic conditions, and cropping patterns have been given due attention. Significant general characteristics of the three zones of Haryana are summarized in Table 4.1, whereas the major attributes of each zone are given below.[4]

The *Northern Region*, including Ambala, Kurukshetra, Karnal, Jind, and Sonepat districts, is a flood plain with some rugged hilly and piedmont terrain, and has a continental climate.

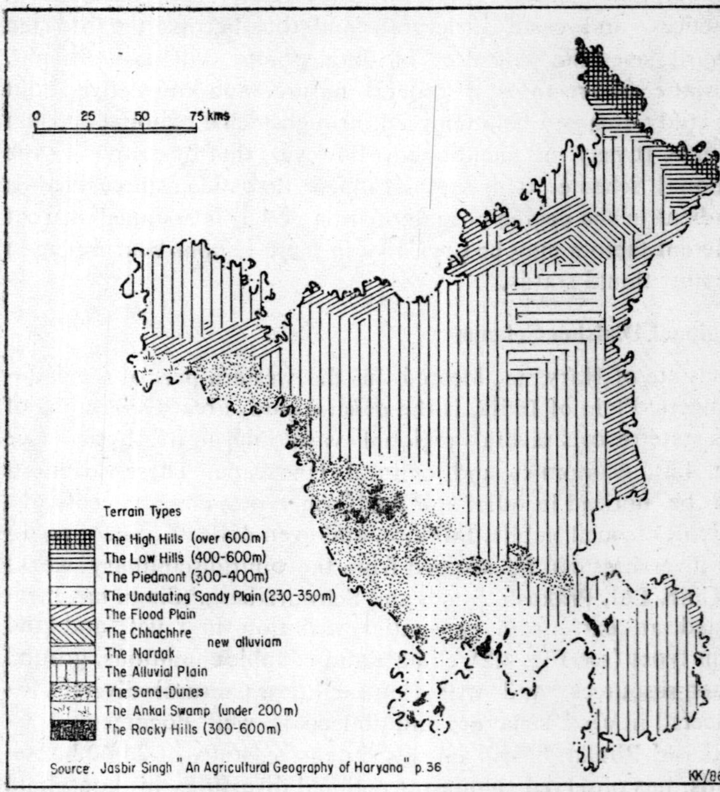


FIG. 4.2 : *Relief and Landform Types in Haryana*

Monsoons and winter cyclones cause most rainfall, which is relatively high in the north: more than 600 mm. With the availability of irrigation facilities, low water deficit, and fertile soils, the region has high agricultural productivity. Wheat and rice are the major food crops, and rural per capita income is highest in this region.

Culturally, this is a Jat (a major farming caste) dominant region with Bangru as the chief spoken dialect. There is a sprinkling of other castes. Participation of Jat and scheduled caste women in the agricultural work-force in this region is high, contrasted with women of other castes. Culturally, breast-feeding

TABLE 4.1 : **Haryana Zonal Division**

| General Characteristics | North | Center | South |
|---|---|---|---|
| Land forms | Mostly plain, some low foot hills of Himalaya, some flood plain | Mostly plain, some sand dunes, narrow flood plain | Undulating plain, low hills, some plain |
| Soil | Alluvial, usually, fertile | Alluvial, light sandy, usually, fertile | Sandy, some new alluvium, usually of low fertility |
| Rainfall | More than 600 mm | 400-600 mm | Less than 400 mm |
| Irrigation: Per cent of net agricultural area | 67 | 55 | 21 |
| Chief food crops | Wheat, rice | Wheat, millets, grains (chick peas) | Millets, wheat |
| Major caste groups | Jats, Rajputs (both farming) | Jats, Bishnoi (both farming) and scheduled castes mostly landless laborers) | Ahirs (farming, pastoral), Jats (farming), Meo/Muslim (pastoral, farming) |
| *Relative* Income Level | High | Intermediate | Low |
| Major food taboos, preferences | Mostly flesh avoidance, use of poultry increasing among Sikh Jats | Mostly flesh avoidance, especially Bishnois who greatly emphasize milk products | Meos prefer meat. Others avoid flesh. Milk products common |

*Source*: S.K. Aggarwal and S.M. Bhardwaj, "Applied Medical Geography and the Developing World: With a Case Study of Malnutrition," in *Applied Geography*; *Selected Perspectives*, ed. John W. Frazier (Englewood, N.J. : Prentice Hall, 1981).

for longer periods is much more common among Jats than other groups. Consumption of milk and milk products such as ghee (clarified butter) and lassi (buttermilk) is usually higher among Jats and Rajputs than other castes.

The *Central Region* comprising Sirsa, Hissar, and Rohtak district (except Jhajjar tehsil), is primalily an alluvial flat plain with a minor concentration of sand dunes in the southern and western parts of Sirsa and Hissar districts, respectively. Annual rainfall is low (400 mm-600 mm) and annual water deficit is high. Net irrigated area is about 55 per cent. The light soils and low precipitation provide a less productive agricultural base than the Northern Region. Wheat, gram (chick peas), and bajra (a millet) are the major staples. Annual household income in this region is lower than in the northern zone.

Jats, Bishnois, scheduled castes, and Jat Sikhs (concentrated in the Sirsa district) constitute the major caste groups of the region. Jats, forming the major cultivator group, are similar in food habits to their counterparts in the northern zone, except for the high emphasis on milk and milk products, and bajra and gram as staples. Bishnois (vegetarians), highly concentrated in Hissar and Sirsa districts, form a distinct cultural group. In their diet, great emphasis is given to the milk products. The average meal is considered incomplete if a milk product is not included in it. Per capita milk consumption in some households reaches as high as half gallon a day. Breast or buffalo milk constitutes the major food of young children.

The *Southern Region* includes Bhiwani, Jhajjar tehsil of Rohtak district, Gurgaon, and Mahendargarh districts. In its physical, economic, and cultural pattern, this is the most diverse zone. The eastern section, covering most of Gurgaon district, is primarily an alluvial plain with protuberations of Aravalli outliers. The central part, consisting of Mahendragarh district and Jhajjar tehsil, is an undulating sandy plain, with intrusions of Aravalli hills in the southern part. The remaining zone, covering most of Bhiwani district, is a sand dune infested area. Because of physiographic complexity and geographic continuity, the above subzones have been grouped in this region (see Fig. 4.1). Net irrigated area is lowest (21%) as compared to other regions. With a poor physical resource base and few irrigation facilities, agriculture in this region is handicapped, aside from few pockets in Gurgaon district and Jhajjar tehsil. The household income is also lowest of the three regions.

Culturally, this region is a mosaic of three predominant castes living in three ecological niches. Ahirs concentrate in the central part; Meos (Muslims), Brahmins, and Rajputs, in the eastern zone; and Jats and scheduled castes (formally called untouchables) in the western zone.

**Selection of Villages**

The malnutrition data were collected in ten specially selected villages from the three zones described above. The villages were selected so as to reflect a gradient in the level of socio-economic conditions, varied physical conditions, and accessibility to health care facilities within the delineated zones. To represent cultural variation, the caste factor was also considered such that each village was typical of the caste structure of the region in consideration. In selection of the villages, village directories and the government officials working at the village level (such as paramedical staff) were consulted. The selection process was heuristic and the intent remained to represent the diversified aspects of each zone. The distinguishing characteristics of each village are given in Appendix A. Although a larger sample of villages could have been more representative of the varied ecological conditions of Haryana, the realities of time (12 weeks), and limited funds available constrained this possibility. Moreover, due to the time constraint, it was not feasible to operationalize this kind of study in several villages without adequate rapport with the local population. By including fewer villages, a closer contact, confidence, and rapport could be established, and, therefore, more reliable and accurate data could be generated. Such a strategy is desirable in a traditional society as the extraction of information is a very cumbersome process. With this in mind, three villages from each ecological zone were chosen and studied intensively. In the south zone, four villages were selected (instead of three) so as to adequately represent the caste structure in the area. In general, the selected villages may not represent a statistical sample of the villages of Haryana. The villages, of course, show the most pronounced ecological conditions prevalent in different parts of the state. An exhaustive sample of the families from these villages is preferred to include most socio-economic and cultural groups of the state.

**Selection of the Families/Respondents**

The number of families from each location depended on the size of the selected village. On the average, nearly 25 per cent of the families had 6-36 months age-group children, and a 50 per cent random sample of these families was used in selection of the respondents. By choosing one child from each family a total of 302 young children were included in the studied sample. In case a family was not available in the village, the alternative child was chosen randomly from the remaining sample. A 50 per cent sample basically represented most socio-economic and cultural groups of the studied villages.

## SELECTION OF THE NUTRITIONAL STATUS INDICATORS

For direct assessment and grading of nutritional status, several measures are available and used. These include clinical signs, biochemical tests, dietary standards, and anthropometry. Due to inherent limitations in each method, an accurate assessment of nutritional status is a matter of degree in accuracy rather than inadequacy.

Clinical signs such as edema, depigmentation of hair and skin, hair strength and sparsity and dermatitis exhibit clear syndromes of nutritional deficiencies.[5] The observer's subjectivity in identification, difficulty in quantification, and late appearance in the course of the disease often limits accuracy. Hence, these observations need to be supplemented by other data. The above limitations, prohibited the use of such methods in this study.

Biochemical tests, which require a sample of blood or urine on the sample population, are one of the most accurate and reliable measures. Field difficulties in collection of samples due to antagonism of the parents, problems of interpretation, and ancillary costs restricts their use to small samples which are examined by professional analysts.

Dietary surveys have been extensively used by the researchers for measuring the caloric and other nutrients intake. The limitations of these surveys in the developing societies have already been discussed in the literature review chapter on India, under the "Problem of Assessment" section. In a traditional society such as India, and particularly in the rural areas, different methods of food preparation, unaccountability of the frequency and quantity of food consumed and seasonality in food habits presents a high risk in dependability of this method.

For rapid and extensive community or regional surveys, anthropometry has been widely suggested as the most helpful method of assessing different degrees and forms of PCM in early childhood.[6] Anthropometry involves somatic measurements such as height, weight, mid-arm circumference, head circumference and skinfold thickness, and comparing them with some standard reference. This method also has advantages and disadvantages. Advantages include: (*i*) ease of operation, (*ii*) less antagonism from parents, (*iii*) simplicity of apparatus, and (*iv*) high correlation with degree of malnutrition measured by other methods.[7] On the other hand, disadvantages encountered are: (*i*) lack of good local standard as reference, (*ii*) need for well trained personnel using standardized conditions and procedures, and (*iii*) need for accurate age. Realizing the advantages, and also at the advice of pediatric experts in India,[8] anthropometry was preferred in assessing the nutritional status of the sampled children.

Weight for age was considered the viable parameter for measuring the nutritional status since most anthropometric studies have preferred it for infants and young children.[9] Other parameters such as weight for height (representing acute energy under-nutrition), height for age[10] (representing more chronic protein energy under-nutrition) and mid-arm circumference are also suggested; however, lack of consensus on precise grading of PCM based on such parameters restricts their use to experimental purposes only. The problem of getting accurate age from the mothers was realized; however, it was resolved by using local references such as important fairs, celestial events, local calendars, and religious festivals. Moreover, the author's acquaintance with the local dialects helped in extracting the accurate information. Mothers were most confident in telling age for the youngest child, while some guessing was involved in the older siblings. Follow up questions helped in ascertaining the accurate

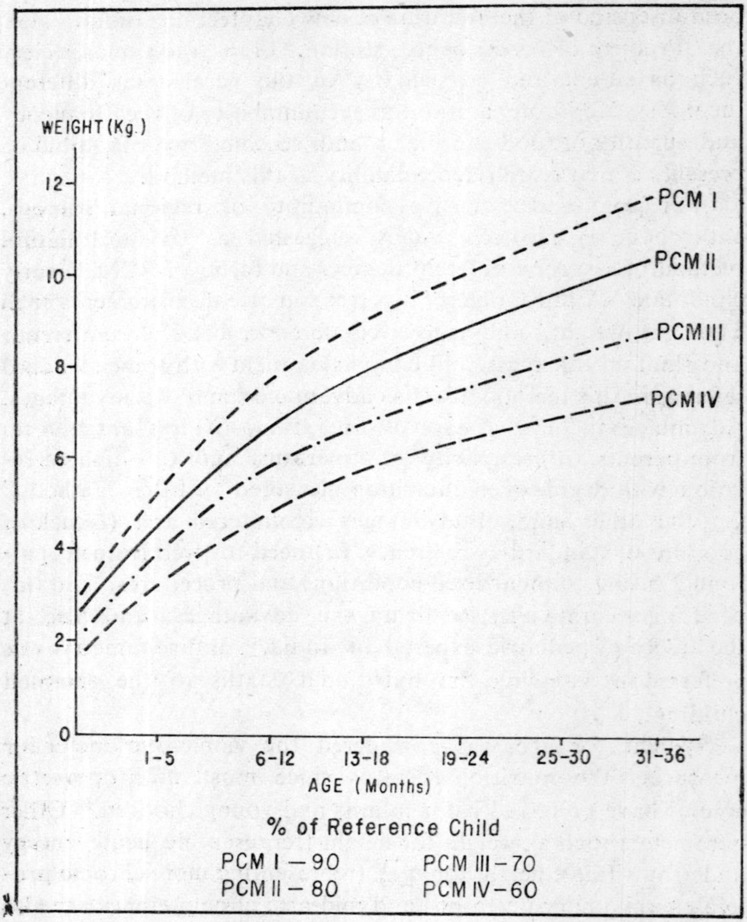


FIG. 4.3 : *Weight Curve from Birth to 3 Years of Age*

age. In measuring weight, the Salter Scales were used and children were weighed as light clothes as admissible through the prevalent standards.

On the basis of weight for age, the nutritional status of each child was graded into four categories of malnutrition (PCM I, PCM II, PCM III, PCM IV).[11] This classification scheme was adopted from the growth chart prepared by the Department of

Social and Preventative Medicine, Medical College, Rohtak, Haryana, using local reference (see Fig. 4.3). The prevalence pattern of PCM in different socio-economic groups and across the studied villages is illustrated in the following chapter.

**Administering the Questionnaire**

The questionnaire for the field work was designed to assess the prevalence of malnutrition among the young children and to determine the functional relationship of various determinants of malnutrition with the nutritional status (see Appendix B). Care was taken in structuring the questionnaire such that information on the most possible direct or indirect causes of malnutrition, as conceptualized earlier, could be generated on each sampled child. The questionnaire was pre-tested and little modification was needed in its instrumentation.[12]

Although the questionnaire was basically administered by the author, the help of the paramedical staff or the headman of the village, who often accompanied the author, was sought in extracting information from the parents of the child. The survey was conducted during the winter months of January to March of 1978. Realizing that malnutrition problem varies from season to season, the prevalence of PCM might have been different if the study was conducted during the summer months. It may be noted that the food availability in rural areas is usually low and the incidence of gastroenteritis infections is often high during the summer. The time and financial constraints prohibited the longitudinal survey of this nature. A further research is suggested in this area.

**Method of Analysis**

Three primary steps are involved in analyzing the malnutrition problem. The first consists in preliminary assessment of the nutritional status. Using weight for age parameter and the PCM classification scheme, different degrees of PCM will be assessed in the sampled population across selected villages and socio-economic groups. Target groups for planned intervention will be identified using cut off points and "trigger levels". Considering the usual practice, 70 per cent weight for age has been chosen as the cut off point for malnourished children. The second step involves the choice of the statistical package for analyzing the survey data on functional relationships.

**Choice of the Multiple Classification Analysis Model**

Among the battery of multivariate techniques which handle this type of problem, the Multiple Classification Analysis (MCA)[13] method was deemed most appropriate due to the following reasons: (1) Since the collected data on most variables in the present study is of a categorical nature (nominal, interval and ordinal level measurements), the traditional multivariate methods were considered less efficient as compared to MCA. The predictors in the MCA model are treated as sets of classes or categories, so it does not matter whether a particular set represents a nominal scale, an ordinal scale, or an interval scale. Moreover, an ordering of scale does not matter in reading the sings of the relations with the dependent variable. (2) MCA program can handle weak measurement (including nominal scale) on the predictor variables, correlated predictors, and non-linear relationships. (3) Basically, it is a multiple regression using dummy variables.[14] Its chief advantage over conventional dummy variable regression is more convenient input arrangement and understandable output that focuses on sets of predictors, and on the extent and direction of the adjustments made for intercorrelations among the sets of predictors. (4) MCA coefficients are all expressed as adjustments to the grand mean, not deviation from the single class which must be excluded from each set when dummy variables are used. Because of this improvement, the regression coefficients in the MCA model are easy to compare and methodologically more accurate. (5) MCA has the ability to show the effect of each predictor on the dependent variable before and after taking into account the effect of all other variables.

In essence, MCA answers two questions: the first question pertains to the closeness of association (relationships) or the proportion of variation in Y that is explained by the variables, and the second question is how the means of the dependent variable (nutrition status) differ between the various classes (such as occupation) of the predictors.

It gives essentially a profile of means of Y over the categories of $X_i$. The statistical model which the program uses is neither new nor complex. The model specifies that a coefficient be assigned to each category of each predictor, and that each person's (or other unit's) score on the dependent variable be treated as sum of the coefficients assigned to categories characterizing them, *plus* the average for all cases, *plus* an error term.

Statistical form of the model as given by Andrews *et al.*, is as follows:

$$Y_{ij} \ldots n = \bar{y} + A_i + B_j + \ldots e_{ij} \ldots n$$

where

$Y_{ij} \ldots n$ = the score (on the dependent variable) of individual $n$ who falls in category $i$ of predictor $A$, category $j$ of predictor $B$, etc.

$\bar{y}$ = grand mean on the dependent variable.

$A_i$ = the "effect" of membership in the $i$th category of predictor $A$.

$B_j$ = the "effect" of membership in the $j$th category of predictor $B$.

$e_{ij} \ldots n$ = error term for this individual.

The main statistics of the program include the number of cases, adjusted and unadjusted class means, adjusted and unadjusted deviations (coefficients) from the grand mean, eta and beta coefficients for each variable, and multiple adjusted and unadjusted coefficients of determination (eta square and beta square respectively). Tests of significance are also included for each variable and for the fitness of the model. The results of the analysis are shown in Chapter 6.

The third step involves identifying the relationship of N.S. with the said determinants at the village level. Since the number of observations is not enough to execute MCA at the village level, a simple correlation technique (Spearman Rank Correlation) has been preferred. The method is not as rigorous as MCA; however, the identified functional relationships will give us fair understanding of the behavior of the associated variables at different locations.

## REFERENCES

1. Chib, Sukhdev Singh, *This Beautiful India: Haryana* (New Delhi: Light and Life Publishers, 1977); Muni Lal, *Haryana on High Road to Prosperity* (Delhi: Vikas Publishing House, 1974); Budha Prakash, *Haryana Through the Ages* (Kurukshetra, India: Kurukshetra University Press, 1970); Jasbir Singh, *An Agricultural Geography of Haryana* (Kurukshetra, India: Vishal Publications, 1976); Joseph E. Schwartzberg, "The Distribution of Selected Castes in the North Indian Plain," *The Geographical Review* 55 (1965).
2. Bhalla, G.S., *Changing Agrarian Structure in India: A Study of the Impact of Green Revolution in Haryana*, Delhi: Meenakshi Prakashan, 1974).
3. In delimiting the three zones, Bhall's scheme has been adopted. See G.S. Bhalla, *Changing Agrarian Structure*, p. 9.
4. The regional description is based substantially on information in Jasbir Singh, *An Agricultural Geography of Haryana.*
5. Swaminathan, M., *Essentials of Food and Nutrition*, Vol. II (Madras: Ganesh & Co., 1974), 307-9.
6. See for example, Ghai, O.P. and Vimlesh Seth, "Grading of Protein Calorie Malnutrition," *Indian Pediatric*, 9 (December 1972), 727-31; E.F.P. Jelliffee and M. Gurney, "Definition of the Problem," in *Nutrition and Malnutrition: Identification and Measurement*, ed., Alex F. Roche and Frank Falkner (London: Plenum Press, 1974), pp. 1-14.
7. Lowenstein, Mathew S. and James F. Phillips, "Evaluation of Arm Circumference Measurement for Determining Nutritional Status of Children and Its Use in an Acute Epidemic of Malnutrition: Owerri, Nigeria, Following the Nigerian Civil War." *The American Journal of Clinical Nutrition* 26 (February 1973), 226-33; A.A. Kanawati, D.S. McLaren, "Mid-Arm/Head Circumference Ratio: A New Technique to assess Marginal Protein-Calorie Malnutrition in a Community," in *Proceedings of the First Asian Congress on Nutrition*, Hyderabad, India, 1972, pp. 786-89.
8. Special mention may be made here of Dr. O.P. Ghai, at the All India Medical Institute, Delhi, and Dr. P. Vasudeva at Medical College, Rohtak, Haryana.
9. Robinow, Meinhard and D.B. Jelliffe, Intercorrelations between Anthropometric Variables. A Contribution to Nutrition Anthropometry of Infancy and Early Childhood in Developing Countries," *Proceedings of the Seventh International Congress of Nutrition*, Vol. 4 (Toronto: Pergamon Press, 1966), pp. 144-47, O.P. Ghai, "Assessment of Protein Calorie Malnutrition," *Indian Pediatrics* 12 (1975), 60-67.
10. Measurements on height were also performed for comparing stature growth in different socio-economic group children; however, its relationship with the N.S. is not attempted in this study.

11. Grades are referred here in terms of percentages: Grade I: 81-90 per cent of the reference weight; Grade II: 71-80 per cent of the reference weight; Grade III: 61-70 per cent of the reference weight. For detailed discussion on grading method see D.B. Jelliffe, *The Assessment of Nutrition Status of Communities* (Geneva: World Health Organization, 1966).
12. For example, questions such as preference given to the child in supply of super foods, fear of osterization by using non-vegetarian foods, wastage in handling of crops were dropped either due to uniformity or a lot of guessing involved in replies.
13. For details see Andrews *et al.*, *Multiple Classification Analysis*.
14. In a dummy variable model, the regression coefficients are derived as deviations from an excluded category coefficient (constrained to zero) of each variable. Therefore, the values of the co-efficients are biased to the number of cases in the excluded category, whereas in the MCA model such a bias is reduced by adjusting the co-efficients in proportion to the number of cases in each category. Moreover, the coefficients are expressed as deviations from the grand mean, in which they are easily understood. For a detailed discussion on deriving the coefficients in both models, the reader is referred to Frank M. Andrews *et al.*, *Multiple Classification Analysis*.

# 5

# Initial Assessment of Nutrition Problem in Haryana

NUTRITION is one of the major factors closely associated with the physical and mental growth of young children. Studies have long shown that nutritional disorders during the crucial period of early childhood lead to growth retardation which might produce residual effects in later years. Therefore, assessing the growth pattern of young children in different geographic units, biological groups (age and sex), and across socio-economic and cultural sections of the community becomes the first step in estimating their nutritional needs. Such an assessment can help in identifying the target groups which need planned intervention for improvement in the N.S.

The growth pattern is analyzed with the assumption that the mean weight in different age-groups should increase in a manner that is expected according to the established regional or national standards. The plotting of such mean weights in relation to the standards (see Fig. 4.3) will thus reflect the deviations in the growth pattern at various locations (villages or zones) and across socio-economic groups. The prevalence of malnutrition will be estimated by classifying the weight deficit of each child in the established categories of PCM. Basically, the intent of this analysis is to assess the prevalence rather than the causes of the malnutrition problem. The later concern is the focus of the succeeding chapter.

While comparing the growth pattern of 302 children, two findings emerge as significant from Fig. 5.1. First, the sampled children, in general, seem to have higher nutritional status than their counterparts in the nation but lower than the expected norm, and significantly lower than the Harvard Standard. Second, the gap between actual and standard weight increases with the advancing age suggesting higher prevalence of PCM in the older age-group children.

**Village Level Assessment**

The weights of 302 children, aggregated at six-month intervals, are presented in Table 5.1. Growth analysis at six-month aggregations will help in identifying age-specific target groups and also the dietary changes associated with age. Fig. 5.2 illustrates growth of sampled children in relation to healthy children (top curve) and malnourished children (bottom curve), across the surveyed villages.

Regional variations in growth pattern of the children are difficult to discern from a small sample of the selected villages. This is indeed a limitation of the study. But, broadly, children located in the physiographically problematic areas (such as sandy, rock terrain of limited agricultural value) showed relatively poor growth, whereas those located in fertile alluvial terrain (such as Mehra, Chandi, Pirthala) had better growth.

At the village level, children of Chandi, Mehra, Landheri, and Firozpur Namak showed better growth pattern than their age-mates in other villages. In these villages the average weights for most age-group children did not deviate much from the standard weight curve. The best nutrition standards were identified in Chandi, where the average weights in all age categories remained higher than those of the region, considerably higher than the national mean, and close to 90 per cent of the reference standard (see Table 5.1). The village had a special advantage of having the Applied Nutrition Program (named "*Aanganwari*") for the pre-school children, sponsored by the Government of Haryana. The availability of nutritious food and an immunization facility through the program probably contributed towards the better health of this village's children.

Firozpur Namak, although located in an economically depressed part of the state, had moderately nourished children in all but two age-groups (Fig. 5.2). Without resorting to a detailed explanation at this point, the typical non-vegetarian food habit pattern of the households and wide coverage of the

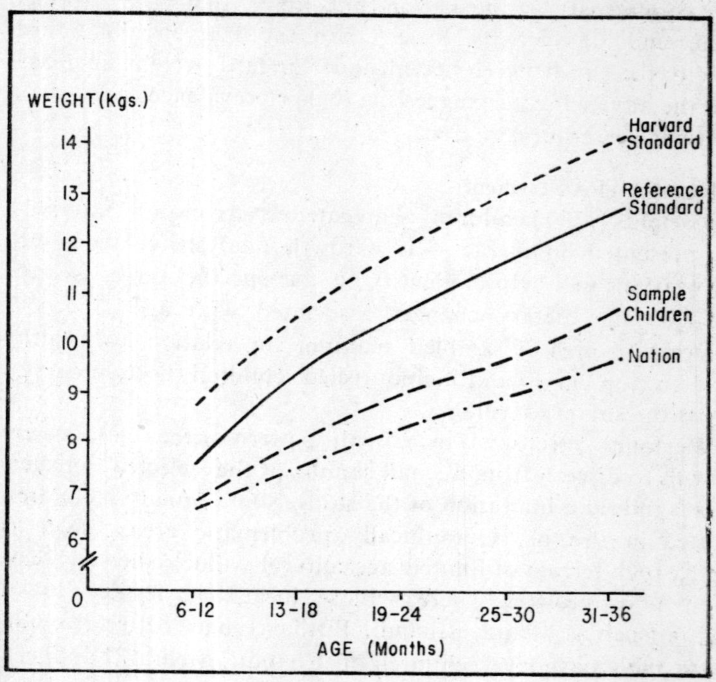


FIG. 5.1 : *Somatic Growth of the Sampled Children*

*Source:* 1. National means calculated from Table 21 in Indian Council of Medical Research, *Studies on Pre-School Children*, ICMR Technical Report Series No. 26, New Delhi, p. 44.
2. Sample children means are calculated by the author from the collected data on children's weight.
3. Reference standard means calculated from the Age-Weight graph after adjusting the 90th percentile for the 100th percentile weight (see Fig. 4.3).
4. Harvard Standard means derived from D.B. Jelliffe *Child Nutrition in the Developing Countries* (Washington, D.C.: Government Printing Office, 1969), 173.

child immunization program probably contributed to the better health of most surveyed children.

The village of Mehra also showed moderate growth pattern except in the first and last age-groups (Table 5.1). Although the impact of the Green Revolution was most noticeable here

TABLE 5.1: **Spatial Variation in the Mean Weights of Sampled Children**

| Age Group (months) | N | North Zone Villages | | | North Zone n=89 | Central Zone Villages | | | Central Zone n=138 |
|---|---|---|---|---|---|---|---|---|---|
| | | Manakpur | Mehra | Sangatpura | | Salamkhera | Landheri | Chandi | |
| 6-12 | 61 | 7.16<br>•(1.44) | 6.23<br>(0.68) | 5.97<br>(1.40) | 6.49<br>(1.29) | 6.74<br>(0.83) | 6.67<br>(1.10) | 6.70<br>(0.14) | 6.69<br>(0.96) |
| 13-18 | 82 | 8.26<br>(2.20) | 8.00<br>(0.90) | 6.99<br>(1.84) | 7.87<br>(1.55) | 7.58<br>(1.68) | 8.99<br>(0.35) | 8.14<br>(0.93) | 8.15<br>(1.30) |
| 19-24 | 37 | 8.10<br>(1.31) | 10.78<br>(3.88) | 9.10<br>(0.01) | 9.38<br>(2.78) | 9.00<br>(1.95) | — | 9.67<br>(2.20) | 9.36<br>(2.02) |
| 25-30 | 77 | 9.64<br>(1.02) | 9.85<br>(1.04) | 10.60<br>(2.23) | 9.93<br>(1.32) | 10.00<br>(1.68) | 9.33<br>(1.06) | 10.12<br>(2.07) | 9.83<br>(1.64) |
| 31-36 | 45 | 8.84<br>(2.39) | 10.70<br>(2.23) | 10.66<br>(1.04) | 10.02<br>(2.02) | 10.15<br>(0.15) | 10.00<br>(1.66) | 11.43<br>(1.81) | 10.91<br>(1.57) |

*(Contd.)*

TABLE 5.1 (*Contd.*)

| Age Group (months) | Pirthala | South Zone Villages | | | South Zone n=105 | Region[1] =302 | Reference Standard Mean Weight[2] | National Mean[3] |
|---|---|---|---|---|---|---|---|---|
| | | Firozpur Namak | Sarangwas | Rajgarh | | | | |
| 6-12 | 6.99 | 7.40 | 7.70 | 6.37 | 7.12 | 6.79 | 7.50 | — |
| | (1.16) | (1.30) | (0.52) | (1.15) | (1.15) | | | |
| 13-18 | 8.33 | 7.47 | 8.34 | 8.01 | 8.07 | 8.03 | 9.44 | 7.55 |
| | (1.15) | (2.03) | (1.10) | (0.70) | (1.28) | | | |
| 19-24 | 9.10 | 8.60 | 8.05 | 8.80 | 8.42 | 9.01 | 10.63 | 8.25 |
| | (1.2) | (0.00) | (2.12) | (2.17) | (1.82) | | | |
| 25-30 | 9.84 | 10.11 | 9.01 | 8.30 | 9.31 | 9.70 | 11.64 | 9.20 |
| | (1.84) | (1.62) | (0.87) | (1.03) | (1.53) | | | |
| 31-36 | 9.97 | 12.05 | 11.68 | 11.50 | 11.30 | 10.76 | 12.64 | 9.75 |
| | (1.18) | (1.85) | (1.75) | (0.42) | (1.63) | | | |

*Entries in Parantheses indicate ± Standard Deviation.

(–) Data Not Available.

1. Region mean calculated after averaging village values in each age-group.
2. Reference standard mean weights calculated from the age-weight graph (see Fig. 4.3).
3. National mean calculated from Table 21 in Indian Council of Medical Research, Studies on Pre-School Children, ICMR Technical Report Series No. 26 ,New Delhi, 1977, p. 44.

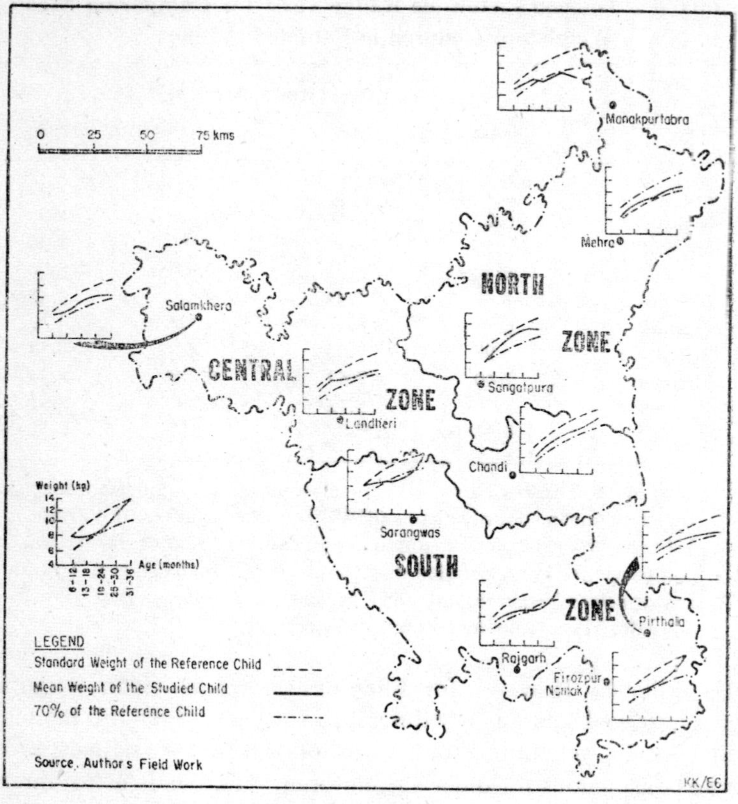


FIG. 5.2 : *Spatial Variation in the Mean Weight of the Sampled Children of Haryana*

(compare irrigated area in Appendix B), the nutrition status was not significantly high as one would expect with the economic growth generated by the Green Revolution. The precise reasons for such variations will be discussed in the following chapter.

In order to ascertain whether the mean weights of the children at different locations are significantly different or not, Duncan's Multiple Range test was performed. The summary results are shown in Table 5.2. Considering all age-groups together (6-36 months) only Chandi children showed significantly higher weights as compared to their counterparts in

TABLE 5.2: **Duncan's Multiple Range Test[1] for Comparing Mean Weights of Children in Sampled Villages**

| Village | Age Group (Months) | | | |
|---|---|---|---|---|
| | 6-12 | 6-24 | 25-36 | 6-36 |
| Manakpur | 7.16 | 7.81 | 9.36* | 8.39 |
| Mehra | 6.23 | 8.13* | 10.13 | 8.80 |
| Sangatpura | 5.93 | 6.84* | 10.63 | 8.39 |
| Salamkhera | 6.74 | 7.73 | 10.02 | 8.70 |
| Landheri | 6.67 | 7.44 | 9.51 | 8.31 |
| Chandi | 6.70 | 8.53* | 10.74* | 9.79* |
| Pirthala | 6.99 | 7.82 | 9.90 | 8.54 |
| Firozpur Namak | 7.40 | 7.57 | 10.82* | 8.85 |
| Sarangwas | 7.70 | 8.12* | 10.50 | 8.91 |
| Rajgarh | 6.37 | 7.89 | 9.01* | 8.31 |

1. This method makes pairwise comparisons of *t* population means based on mean sum of squares ($S^2W$) from the Analysis of Variance. Villages with (*) sign are found significantly different in pairwise comparisons. For a detailed discussion on this method, see: Lyman Ott, *An Introduction to Statistical Methods and Data Analysis* (North Scituate, Mass : Duxbury Press, 1977), pp. 392-95.

other villages. However, for different age-groups, mean weights were observed significantly different in at least seven of the ten villages. In general spatial variation in mean weights seems more conspicuous for older age children. That leads us to infer the possibility of varying environmental, cultural, demographic, and health influences in causing such variations.

**Age Specific Assessment**

In age-specific analysis two findings emerge significant from Fig. 5.2. First, the mean weight curves in the young age-group (6-18 months) children are close to the standard weight curve across most villages. This trend may be ascribed to the usual breast-feeding practice in most young mothers. Around 88 per cent of the children below 18 months were reported to be either fully or partially breast-fed. At this stage, the influence of social, economic, cultural, or environmental factors on growth is minimal. Most essential nutrients for growth are normally available from mother's milk.

Second, an unsymmetric growth pattern is noticed for most older age-group children (19-36 months). Except the villages of Chandi and Firozpur Namak, the mean weights in the above age-groups remained below or close to the 70 per cent reference curve. The influence of weaning seems to be operating at this stage. Twenty-five per cent of the children were partially or fully breast-fed and the rest were being weaned or fed on the local foods. Evidently, the exogenous factors, such as unsanitary living conditions and food habits of parents, happen to constrain the availability of essential nutrients in the diet pattern of a child. Furthermore, spatial variation of such factors probably explains the erratic behavior of the mean weight curve after 18 months. The precise influence of the exogenous factors is discussed in the following chapter.

In short, 6-18 months children in the studied villages are relatively healthy, whereas most children in the 19-36 months category are underweight for their age. The spatial variation in mean weights is more pronounced in older age children, whereas variation in the younger age-group is less significant. The erratic behavior in the mean weights is more pronounced in older age children, whereas variation in the younger age-group is less significant. The erratic behavior in the mean weights, particularly after the first year of life, obviously reflects the spatial dimension of the malnutrition problem. Until the age of one, probably due to the universal breast-feeding practice, the nutritional constraints on the food path of the child are minimum, whereas during the later years the spatially varying externalities (social, cultural, economic, and health accessibility factors) become more operative in regulating the food intake and thus the N.S.

## PREVALENCE PATTERN OF PCM AND IDENTIFICATION OF TARGET GROUPS

The preceding analysis portrayed the general nature of the malnutrition problem across villages and specific age-groups. The prevalence pattern of the problem could not be estimated, since the weight deficits/gains were not classified according to the established standards. Using the Jelliffe grading scheme and local standards (see Fig. 4.3), each child was placed in one of

TABLE 5.3: **Prevalence of PCM in the Studied Population**

| Category | Number of Children (Sample) | Per cent Children | Per cent** Children in India | Per cent** Children in Rural Hyderabad |
|---|---|---|---|---|
| Normal* | 30 | 10.06 | 3 | 1.6 |
| Grade I | 69 | 22.84 | 14 | 15.7 |
| Grade II | 91 | 30.13 | 65*** | 34.1 |
| Grade III | 75 | 24.73 | | 34.6 |
| Grade IV | 37 | 12.24 | 18 | 14.1 |

* Normal category includes children with weight greater than 90 per cent of the standard weight.

** Shown for comparison only.

*** Aggregated for Grade II and Grade III.

the four categories of PCM. The prevalence estimates of PCM for the entire population are presented in Table 5.3. For comparative purposes, the prevalence figures are also given for India (although on slightly different classification system) and for the rural area surrounding Hyderabad.

It is apparent from Table 5.3 that around 10 per cent of the sampled children possessed normal health. Even this small proportion of Haryana children in good health is relatively higher than several regional or national estimates.[1]

The most vulnerable group, included in the fourth category, constitutes nearly 12 per cent of the sampled population. Such children, according to most nutrition experts, are listed as marasmus, or marasmic kwashirkor, when edema is also present. Children in categories II and III suffer from a mild to moderate form of PCM, and are referred to as 'underweight' or suffering with 'mass wasting' due to muscle-tissue loss. They constitute more than half of the total surveyed children. Briefly stated, the prevalence of malnutrition of category IV is consistent with the national estimates, whereas in terms of normal health, Haryana children are far ahead of the nation.

The village level prevalence patterns are shown in Table 5.4 and Fig. 5.3. The findings correspond greatly to the earlier mean weight analysis. By aggregating prevalence figures for categories I and II, Mehra, Landheri, Chandi, Firozpur Namak,

TABLE 5.4: **Prevalence of PCM in the Surveyed Villages**

| Village/Nutrition Category | Normal* and PCM I | | PCM II | | PCM III | | PCM IV | |
|---|---|---|---|---|---|---|---|---|
| | N | Per cent | N | Per cent | N | Per cent | N | Per cent |
| Manakpur | 8 | 25.8 | 11 | 35.5 | 6 | 19.4 | 6 | 19.4 |
| Mehra | 8 | 22.2 | 15 | 41.7 | 10 | 27.8 | 3 | 8.3 |
| Sangatpura | 5 | 22.7 | 8 | 36.4 | 5 | 22.7 | 4 | 18.2 |
| Salamkhera | 11 | 31.4 | 9 | 25.7 | 10 | 28.5 | 5 | 14.3 |
| Landheri | 15 | 41.7 | 9 | 25.0 | 8 | 22.2 | 4 | 11.1 |
| Chandi | 15 | 40.5 | 10 | 27.0 | 8 | 21.6 | 4 | 10.8 |
| Pirthala | 8 | 30.8 | 8 | 30.8 | 9 | 34.6 | 1 | 3.8 |
| Firozpur Namak | 14 | 50.0 | 5 | 17.9 | 7 | 25.0 | 2 | 7.1 |
| Sarangwas | 10 | 37.0 | 9 | 33.3 | 6 | 22.2 | 2 | 7.4 |
| Rajgarh | 5 | 20.8 | 7 | 29.2 | 6 | 25.0 | 6 | 25.0 |
| Total Sample | 99 | 32.8 | 91 | 30.1 | 75 | 24.8 | 37 | 12.3 |

*The Normal category has been merged with Category I for analysis purpose. In nutritional terms, both categories are not significantly different and their merger will not influence the results greatly.

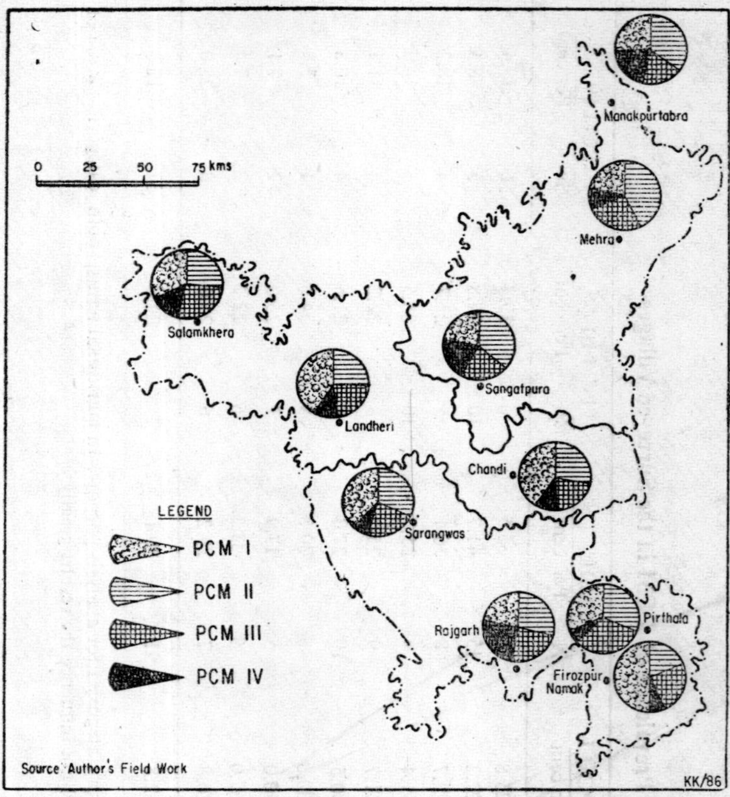


FIG. 5.3 : *Prevalence of Protein Calorie Malnutrition (PCM) in the Sampled Villages of Haryana*

and Sarangwas emanate as having children with moderate to good health.[2] On the other hand, the rest of the five villages had moderately to acutely malnourished children. The villages of Manakpur, Sangatpura in the North Zone, Salamkhera in the Central Zone, and Pirthala and Rajgarh in the South Zone are treated here as target villages and need immediate to long-term nutritional intervention to combat the PCM problem. The critical age-groups along with target villages are highlighted in Table 5.5.

TABLE 5.5: **Target Villages and Age Groups**

| Zone | Village | Prevalence (PCM III, PCM IV) | Age Group (months) |
|---|---|---|---|
| | *MANAKPURTABRA | 38.8 | 19-24; 31-36 |
| North | Mehra | 36.1 | |
| | *SANGATPURA | 40.9 | 6-12; 13-18 |
| | *SALAMKHERA | 42.8 | 31-36 |
| Central | Landheri | 33.3 | |
| | Chandi | 32.4 | |
| | *PIRTHALA | 38.4 | 31-36 |
| South | Firozpur Namak | 32.1 | |
| | Sarangwas | 29.6 | |
| | *RAJGARH | 50.0 | 25-30 |

*These villages contain more than average rate of PCM III and PCM IV for the entire population and are defined here as target villages.

### SOMATIC GROWTH PATTERN IN DIFFERENT SOCIO-ECONOMIC GROUPS

The varied socio-economic conditions identified in the studied households warrant a separate assessment of nutrition status for the different social and economic group children. Such variations were found more pronounced for occupation, caste, and income groups. Moreover, the assessment of nutrition status across such groups will facilitate identifying the target population for more efficient delivery of nutrition programs. With this consideration in mind the following analysis discusses the somatic growth pattern in major socio-economic group children.

### ASSESSMENT OF CHILDREN'S NUTRITION STATUS RELATED TO FAMILY INCOME GROUP

A careful examination of Table 5.6 reveals, with some exceptions, a general increase in mean weights of different age-group children with increase in income. This simple relationship is more clearly portrayed in Fig. 5.4 where children from high income families appear relatively heavier than their counterparts in medium and low income families. An analysis of variance

TABLE 5.6: **Mean Weight of Sampled Children Related with Family Income Group**

(*Weight in Kilogram*)

| Age Group (months) | Less Than Rs. 1200* | Rs. 1201-2400 | Rs. 2401-4800 | Rs. 4801-8400 | Greater than Rs. 8400 | Sample Mean Weight | Reference Standard Mean Weight | Nation Mean Weight |
|---|---|---|---|---|---|---|---|---|
| | n=34 | n=100 | n=74 | n=52 | n=42 | n=302 | | |
| 6-12 | 6.60 | 6.47 | 6.71 | 6.98 | 7.63 | 6.69 | 7.50 | — |
| 13-18 | 5.98 | 8.01 | 8.05 | 8.44 | 8.91 | 8.15 | 9.44 | 7.55 |
| 19-24 | 8.05 | 8.36 | 8.03 | 9.03 | 10.00 | 9.36 | 10.63 | 8.25 |
| 25-30 | 8.86 | 9.13 | 9.91 | 10.08 | 10.90 | 9.83 | 11.64 | 9.20 |
| 31-36 | 8.95 | 11.07 | 10.73 | 11.80 | 11.04 | 10.91 | 12.64 | 9.75 |

*One dollar apyroximates twelue rupees.

*Source:* Author's Field Work.

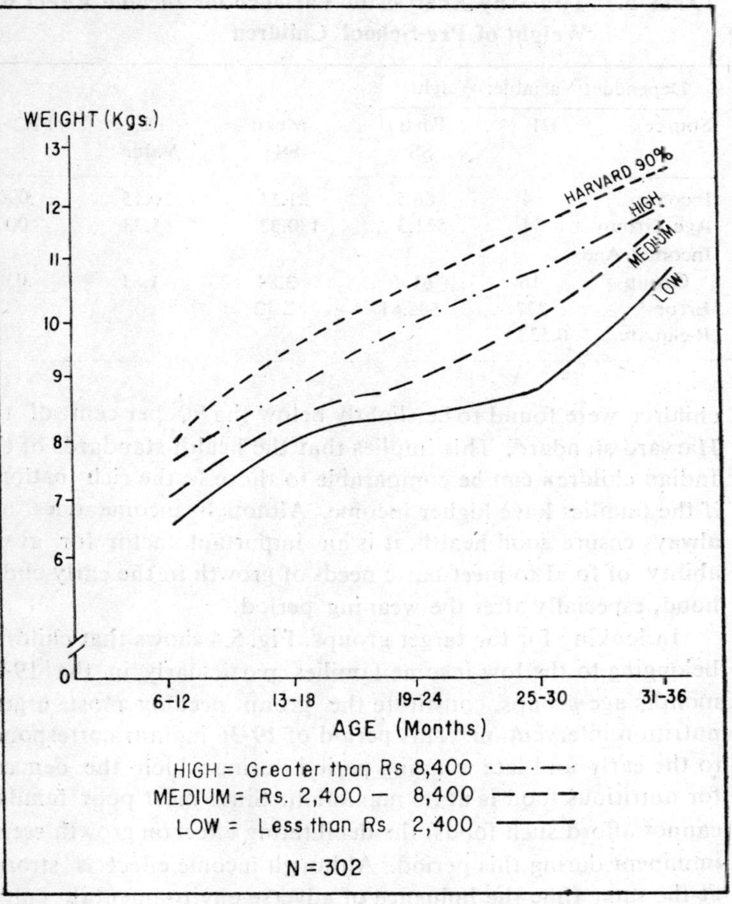


FIG. 5.4 : *Mean Weight of Children—Family's Income Groups*

was also performed in order to validate the statistical significance of the above finding that mean weights are significantly higher for the rich children as compared to the poor. The results in Table 5.7 confirm that the mean weights in different income and age-groups (see income *age-group effect) are significantly different with a PR>.05.

Furthermore, by comparing the growth pattern of rich children with their counterparts in the rich nations, the Haryana

TABLE 5.7: **Two-Way Analysis of Variance for Income Effect on Weight of Pre-School Children**

Dependent Variable: Weight

| Source | DF | Partial SS | Mean SS | F Value | PR>F |
|---|---|---|---|---|---|
| Income | 4 | 86.5 | 21.54 | 10.15 | .0002 |
| Age Group | 4 | 521.3 | 130.32 | 61.33 | ·0001 |
| Income* Age Group | 16 | 61.4 | 3.84 | 1.81 | .03 |
| Error | 277 | 588.61 | 2.12 | | |
| R-Square | 0.532 | | | | |

children were found to be slightly below the 90 per cent of the Harvard standard. This implies that the health standards of the Indian children can be comparable to those in the rich nations, if the families have higher income. Although income does not always ensure good health, it is an important factor for availability of food to meet basic needs of growth in the early childhood, especially after the weaning period.

In looking for the target groups, Fig. 5.4 shows that children belonging to the low income families, particularly in the 19-36 months age-groups, constitute the group needing most urgent nutrition intervention. This period of 19-36 months corresponds to the early and late weaning period during which the demand for nutritious food is at its maximum. Since most poor families cannot afford such foods, the debilitating effect on growth seems imminent during this period. Although income effect is strong, at the same time the influence of adverse environmental, cultural, and demographic factors which, as a matter of fact, could aggravate the low income effect, cannot be minimized.

In prevalence terms, nearly 45 per cent of the low income children suffered from a moderate to severe form of malnutrition (Table 5.8), contrasted with only 19.1 per cent of the rich children. Realizing the large proportion of children under PCM III and PCM IV categories in low income families, income specific nutrition programs deserve attention to combat the malnutrition problem.

TABLE 5.8 : **Prevalence of PCM in Different Income Group Children**

| Annual income (Rs.) | PCM I | | PCM II | | PCM III | | PCM IV | | Total | |
|---|---|---|---|---|---|---|---|---|---|---|
| | n | Per cent | n | Per cent | n | Per cent | n | Per cent | n | Per cent |
| "Low" (Less than 4,800) | 34 | 25.4 | 40 | 29.9 | 35 | 26.1 | 25 | 18.6 | 134 | 44.4 |
| "Medium" (4801-8400) | 44 | 34.9 | 38 | 30.2 | 34 | 27.0 | 10 | 7.9 | 126 | 41.7 |
| "High" (More than 8400) | 21 | 50.0 | 13 | 31.0 | 6 | 14.3 | 2 | 4.8 | 42 | 13.9 |

*Source* : Author's Field Work.

## ASSESSMENT OF NUTRITION STATUS IN DIFFERENT CASTE CHILDREN

A perusal of nutrition literature on India indicates little effort to analyze the nutrition problem from a caste perspective. Rather, most studies emphasise income, sex, age, or locale in differentiating the nutrition status of young children. Nevertheless, caste specific analysis in India's context seems desirable, as castes reflect to a great extent the socio-economic fabric of the society. In nutrition studies such an investigation is even more pertinent, since food habits vary considerably with caste.[3] Due to regional variation of castes in Haryana, it presents an ideal example for investigating nutritional differences across various caste children. Nine major caste groups are identified from the present field survey.[4] By examining the mean weight in Table 5.9, the better nourished children are recorded among the traditionally cultivator caste groups (Jat Sikh, Jat and Rajput, Meo and Bishnoi), and business (Khatri/Arora) castes, whereas less nourished children are observed among the scheduled castes. Children in other groups displayed an irregular growth pattern. For example, children from Brahmin and Vaishya social groups illustrate very poor growth in the first two years and moderate growth thereafter. Similarly, respondents from Ahir and Gujar families portray a good health standard (except in the 13-18 months and 31-36 months age categories). Detailed explanation for such an erratic growth trend is beyond the scope of this chapter. Probably, the small number of observations in each age-group cell might be responsible for disrupting the trend.

A graphic presentation of mean weights and heights of six major castes also demonstrates the varying nature of somatic parameters with caste (Fig. 5.5). Meo children are observed heavier, and Ahir/Gujar children taller than all other castes. Scheduled and artizan castes contained the least developed children. As in income analysis, 6-12 months children showed little variation in the mean weights, whereas the older children (31-36 months) demonstrated a varying growth pattern across different castes. The same is observed to be true for the mean heights. Again, we can say that the younger children, irrespective of their social cultural attributions, are healthy, whereas the

TABLE 5.9 : **Mean Weight of Pre-School Children in Different Castes**

| Age Group (months) | N | Jat Sikhs | Jat Rajputs | Brahmin and Vaishyas | Khatri/ Arora | Meo/ Muslim | Scheduled Castes | Artizan | Bishnoi | Ahir/ Gujars | Region mean weight | Reference standard mean weight | Nation mean weight |
|---|---|---|---|---|---|---|---|---|---|---|---|---|---|
| | | n=12 | n=77 | n=19 | n=33 | n=25 | n=60 | n=38 | n=15 | n=23 | n=302 | | |
| 6-12 | 61 | 6.50 | 6.52 | 5.25 | 7.26 | 7.57 | 6.78 | 6.30 | 7.25 | 6.52 | 6.69 | 7.50 | — |
| 13-18 | 82 | 8.02 | 8.29 | 8.12 | 8.98 | 8.47 | 6.95 | 8.10 | 9.14 | 8.95 | 8.15 | 9.44 | 7.55 |
| 19-24 | 37 | 11.30 | 10.17 | 8.20 | 8.70 | 8.60 | 8.33 | 8.23 | — | 8.12 | 9.36 | 10.63 | 8.25 |
| 25-30 | 77 | 11.30 | 9.98 | 9.63 | 9.67 | 9.92 | 9.05 | 9.30 | 9.70 | 8.90 | 9.83 | 11.64 | 9.20 |
| 31-36 | 45 | — | 10.71 | 11.70 | 11.84 | 12.10 | 9.71 | 9.86 | 9.80 | 11.52 | 10.91 | 12.64 | 9.75 |

*Nation mean weight figures derived by averaging mean weight-figures for boys and girls in Table 21, Indian Council of Medical Research, *Studies on Pre-School Children*, ICMR Technical Report Series No. 26, New Delhi, 1977, p. 44.

TABLE 5.10 : **Analysis of Variance for Comparing Weight of Pre-School Children in Different Castes**

Dependent variable : Weight

| Source | DF | Partial SS | Mean SS | F | PR>F |
|---|---|---|---|---|---|
| Caste | 8 | 76.76 | 9.59 | 4.28 | 0.0001 |
| Age Group | 4 | 513.75 | 128.44 | 57.29 | 0.0001 |
| Caste * Age Group | 30 | 86.34 | 2.88 | 1.28 | 0.1548 |
| Error | 259 | 530.65 | 2.24 | | |
| R-Square | 0.538 | | | | |

older children suffer more as a result of socio-economic conditions.

Although a cursory examination of Table 5.9 and Fig. 5.5 indicates a variance in the nutritional status across various castes, an analysis of variance demonstrated the statistical significance of such variance (see Table 5.10). In identifying the target groups, the prevalence analysis (Table 5.11) denotes a high proportion of scheduled caste (55%), artizan caste (39.5%) and Brahmin and Vaishya caste (52.6%) children as the most vulnerable groups. More than 50 per cent of the malnourished children (adding categories III and IV) belonged to the above castes, whereas they constitute only 39 per cent of the sample population. Obviously, a caste-specific planning strategy is warranted from this analysis, although such a suggestion may have its political reverberations. Nutritional status variations were also noticed across other variables (such as sex, family structure); however, such variations appeared to be insignificant in statistical terms, and hence are not treated in the present discussion.

## Conclusions

In short, the following conclusions can be derived from the preceding analysis:

About one-third of the sampled children showed normal growth, whereas more than one-third had been suffering from moderate to severe form of PCM. In general, the nutrition

TABLE 5.11 : **Prevalence of PCM in Different Caste Children**

| Caste | PCM I | | PCM II | | PCM III | | PCM IV | | N |
|---|---|---|---|---|---|---|---|---|---|
| | n | Per cent | n | Per cent | n | Per cent | n | Per cent | |
| Jat Sikh | 5 | 41.7 | 5 | 43.7 | 1 | 8.3 | 1 | 8.3 | 12 |
| Jat/Rajput | 21 | 27.3 | 33 | 42.9 | 17 | 22.1 | 6 | 7.8 | 77 |
| Brahmin/Vaishya | 5 | 26.3 | 4 | 21.1 | 8 | 42.1 | 2 | 10.5 | 19 |
| Khatri/Arora | 17 | 51.5 | 7 | 21.2 | 6 | 18.2 | 3 | 9.1 | 33 |
| Meo/Muslim | 11 | 44.0 | 5 | 20.0 | 7 | 28.0 | 2 | 8.0 | 25 |
| Scheduled Caste (mostly Harijans) | 11 | 18.3 | 16 | 26.7 | 22 | 36.7 | 11 | 18.3 | 60 |
| Artizan | 9 | 23.7 | 14 | 36.8 | 10 | 26.3 | 5 | 13.2 | 28 |
| Bishnoi | 10 | 66.7 | 2 | 13.3 | 1 | 6.7 | 2 | 13.3 | 15 |
| Ahir/Gujar | 10 | 43.5 | 5 | 21.7 | 3 | 13.0 | 5 | 21.7 | 23 |
| Total | 99 | 32.8 | 91 | 30.1 | 75 | 24.8 | 37 | 12.3 | 302 |

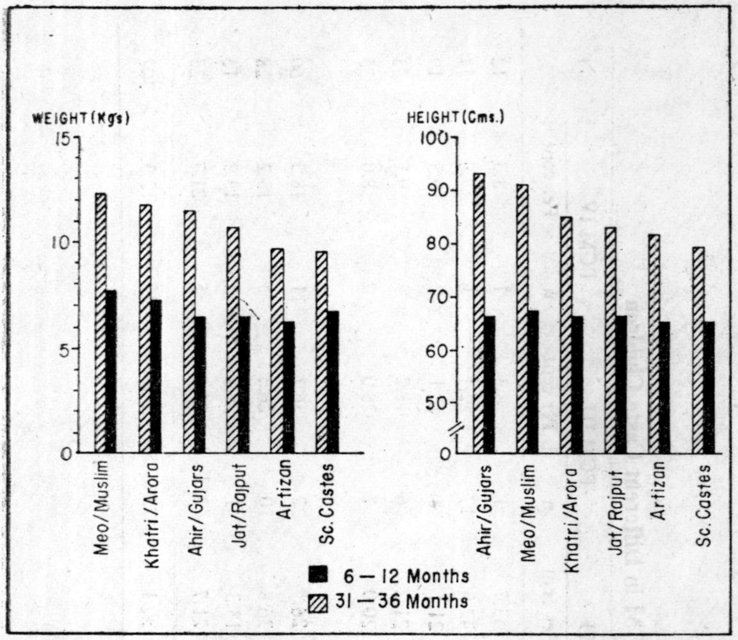


FIG. 5.5 : *Weight and Height Comparison Among Children of Different Castes in Haryana*

status of Haryana children was observed to be relatively higher than that of their counterparts in the nation.

In age-specific assessment, younger children (6-23 months) emerged healthier than the older children (24-36 months). This finding indicates that older children are more vulnerable to nutritional disorders and hence the nutrition programs should be age-specific in their instrumentation and delivery.

In spatial terms, the mean weights of children, in most age-groups, were significantly different across the villages. By comparing the mean weights and prevalence estimates, Chandi, an Applied Nutrition Program village located in an agriculturally developed area, contained the most well nourished children. Contrastingly, the highest proportion (50%) of malnourished children was observed in Rajgarh, a village located in the sand dune and hilly terrain of the South Zone. Inter-village variations of this nature obviously illustrate the varying influence of locational factors (such as food habits, micro-environment, health facilities) on the health status of the sampled subjects. Detailed consequences of such factors are deliberated in the succeeding chapter.

Castewise differences in the mean weights and prevalence pattern were also observed in different age-group children. In general, better nourished children belonged to the cultivator castes, whereas less nourished children had maximum occurrence in scheduled and artizan castes, forming the largest labour group. A high proportion of Brahmin and Vaishya castes children emerged in the low nutrition status category. The finding seems contrary to the general belief that children belonging to the higher castes (with relatively higher income) usually possess good health. It might be interesting to investigate the specific causes which lead to low nutritional status in these higher and lower castes children.

Broadly, children belonging to high income families had less growth problems. Although a significant difference existed in the mean weights across different income group children, the bias was stronger in the higher age-groups. This finding suggests the importance of low income and older age-group oriented applied nutrition programs rather than a blanket approach where such biases are generally ignored.

## REFERENCES

1. Indian Council of Medical Research, p. 51; Gopalan and Raghavan, *Nutrition Atlas of India*, p. 75; Rao *et al.*, "Nutrition Status of Children Around Delhi," p. 1495.
2. Better nourished and malnourished villages are those which have higher prevalence figures than the total sample mean in Table 5.4. The malnourished villages are treated here as "target villages" needing planned intervention to correct nutrition problem.
3. See Chakravarti, "Regional Preferences for Food," pp. 395-410.
4. *Jat Sikh*: Includes farming people of Sikh religion who mostly settled in Northern Haryana after India's Independence. They do not have taboos against meat eating except beef. *Jat and Rajput*: This group includes those Hindu caste people of Haryana whose traditional occupation is farming. Rajput, even though they belong to the warrior caste, traditionally form a farming caste. Both castes are basically vegetarian by preference. Regional concentration in central and

western parts of Haryana. *Brahmin and Vaishya*: This group,although composed of a traditionally 'priestly' caste and a 'trading-commerce' caste, does nevertheless have functionally numerous similarities. Both groups are strict vegetarian by choice. *Khatri and Arora*: These are mostly Punjabi trading Hindu caste settlers who came to Haryana after 1947. At present there is diversity of occupation within this caste group. Irrespective of their income group, most Punjabis observe cleanliness as an established habit. *Meo/Muslim*: Although strictly the Meos of Haryana, being Muslim, should not be considered a caste, in Haryana's social context they have been treated as a caste group for analytical purposes. Culturally, they are more Hinduized, and celebrate some Hindu festivals and perform Hindu rituals for marriage, birth, and death. The major difference from Hindus is in terms of food habits, as meat constitutes a significant portion of their diet. Geographically, they are concentrated in Firozpur Jhirka tehsil of Gurgaon. Their children were observed as one of the most healthy groups due to their food habits and living conditions. *Scheduled Castes*: All castes considered as scheduled (formally called "untouchables") are included in this category. These are Chamaars, Ramadasias, Balmikis, and other such categories. They often work as farm labour or are traditional shoe-makers. Nutrition standard is usually low due to low income and unsanitary living conditions. *Artizan*: This includes variety of jatis whose traditional occupations are weaving cloth (Julaha), carpenter (Tarkhan), Blacksmith (Lohar) and the like. *Bishnoi*: The word derived from 'Vaishnava' literally means "pure vegetarian." Their typical food habits related to vegetarianism and use of milk and milk products distinguishes them as a distinct cultural group. By all standards their children were better nourished than their counterparts in other castes of the region. They are located primarily in the Hissar district. *Ahir and Gujars*: Ahir and Gujars are traditionally cowherders, but at present most of them are cultivators. Ahirs are primarily located in the southern parts of Haryana.

# 6

# Determinants of Malnutrition

THE assessment analysis in the preceding chapter clearly demonstrates that a malnutrition problem exists with varying severity at different locations, and among various socio-economic group children. The demonstration of association of a disease with place implies that some etiological factors are present in the family or local ecology of the affected areas. In the conceptualization some possible determinants which influence or are associated with the malnutrition problem are already outlined. In brief, the effort at this point is to assess the functional relationship of those determinants in explaining the varying behavior of the nutritional status of the sampled children.

In estimating such relationships, the Multiple Classification Analysis model, as described in Chapter 4, has been used. The basic form of our model is as follows:

NS=f (dependent variable) {
Infection Tendency of the Child
Quality of Living Environment
Family Annual Income
Size of Family
Birth Interval
Food Group
Work Status of Mother
Occupation of the Head of Household
} Independent Variables[1]

The model will help us in answering four questions pertaining to the strength of individual variables and their combined effect in explaining the nutritional status variation of the sampled population:[2]

(1) Do all the variables "together explain a significant" portion of the variance of the dependent variables? This will be examined by the $F_1$ test.
(2) Does this variable "all by itself explain a significant portion of the variance of the dependent variable?" This will be tested by the $F_2$ test.
(3) Does this independent variable "explain a significant portion of the variance of the dependent variable over and above that which can be explained by the other predictors?" This will be assessed by the $F_3$ test.
(4) Would this independent variable "explain a significant portion of the variance of the dependent variable if we would hold constant the other predictors?" This will be evaluated by the $F_4$ test.

Further, along with predictors' effect, the model also computes the category-effect of each variable in explaining the NS variation. By comparing the coefficient means across different categories of a variable, we can ascertain what sub-group of the sample has been influenced most or least in their NS by different variables in the model. This can help us in identifying the critical groups needing interventions.

## ANALYSIS OF THE DETERMINANTS OF MALNUTRITION

Before discussing the individual determinants, a general analysis for the entire model reveals that the eight included variables explained a significant portion of variation of the dependent variable (see $F_1$ test in Table 6.1). Among the individual variables, only Quality of Living Environment did not explain a significant amount of variance when considered with other variables ($F_4$ test), whereas its importance did not decline when treated in bivariate relationship. All other variables emerged as significant explanators of N.S. both in bivariate and multivariate

TABLE 6.1: **Predictors by their Importance in Explaining the Nutritional Status of the Haryana Children**

| Predictors | Coefficients | | Eta² | Beta² | Significant Tests | | | No. of Cases | Per cent Malnourished |
|---|---|---|---|---|---|---|---|---|---|
| | Unadjusted | Adjusted | | | $F_2$ | $F_3$ | $F_4$ | | |
| 1 | 2 | 3 | 4 | 5 | 6 | 7 | 8 | 9 | 10 |
| *Infection Tendency* | | | .0840 | .0537 | 13.713* | 23.281* | 10.685* | | |
| Low | −0.3053 | −0.2356 | | | | | | 93 | 23.7 |
| Medium | −0.1105 | −0.0983 | | | | | | 109 | 33.1 |
| High | 0.4044 | 0.3263 | | | | | | 100 | 54.0 |
| *Quality of Micro-Environment* | | | .0603 | .0044 | 9.588* | 1.924 | 0.883 | | |
| Very Good | −0.5794 | −0.1717 | | | | | | 29 | 13.7 |
| Satisfactory | −0.1080 | −0.215 | | | | | | 139 | 35.2 |
| Poor | 0.2374 | 0.0595 | | | | | | 134 | 44.0 |
| *Family Annual Income* | | | .0682 | .0424 | 5.435* | 9.187* | 4.216* | | |
| Rs. 0-1200 | 0·5697 | 0.4363 | | | | | | 34 | 61.8 |
| Rs. 1201-2400 | 0.0944 | 0.524 | | | | | | 100 | 39.0 |
| Rs. 2401-4800 | 0.0169 | 0.317 | | | | | | 94 | 39.2 |
| Rs. 4801-8400 | −0.1848 | −0.1395 | | | | | | 52 | 28.9 |
| Rs. 8401 and above | −0.4274 | −0.3611 | | | | | | 42 | 19.1 |

(*Contd.*)

TABLE 6.1 (*Contd.*)

| 1 | 2 | 3 | 4 | 5 | 6 | 7 | 8 | 9 | 10 |
|---|---|---|---|---|---|---|---|---|---|
| *Birth Interval* | | | .0350 | .0281 | 3.595* | 8.121* | 3.737* | | |
| 18 months and below | 0.2233 | 0.1773 | | | | | | 18 | 38.9 |
| 19-36 months | 0.1265 | 0.1201 | | | | | | 178 | 42.7 |
| 37 months and above | −0.1831 | −0.2316 | | | | | | 57 | 26.3 |
| Only child | −0.3288 | −0.2318 | | | | | | 49 | 28.6 |
| *Number of Children* | | | .0484 | .0120 | 4.593* | 9.366 | 4.299 | | |
| Two or less | −0.2673 | −0.1634 | | | | | | 124 | 28.2 |
| Three-Four | −0.0344 | −0.0885 | | | | | | 118 | 36.4 |
| Five and above | 0.3256 | 0.3478 | | | | | | 60 | 56.7 |
| *Food Group of the Child* | | | .0570 | .0196 | 6.008* | 5.645* | 2.580* | | |
| Protein Dominant | 0.0147 | 0.0248 | | | | | | 122 | 35.2 |
| Carbohydrate Dominant | 0.4618 | 0.2607 | | | | | | 51 | 60.8 |
| Mixed (Protein and Carb.) | −0.1369 | −0.0961 | | | | | | 105 | 31.5 |
| Balanced | −0.4572 | −0.2598 | | | | | | 24 | 20.8 |

| | | | | | | | | | |
|---|---|---|---|---|---|---|---|---|---|
| *Work Status of Mother* | | | .0164 | .0198 | 4.996* | 17.148* | 7.871* | | |
| Works | 0.1394 | 0.1532 | | | | | | 141 | 44.7 |
| Does not work | −0.1221 | −0.1342 | | | | | | 161 | 30.4 |
| *Occupation of Head of Household* | | | .0421 | .0298 | 3.266* | 6.455* | 2.962* | | |
| Less than 10 Acres | −0.0781 | −0.2354 | | | | | | 80 | 35.5 |
| 11-30 Acres | −0.2766 | −0.1646 | | | | | | 36 | 25.0 |
| 31 and Above | −0.1655 | 0.3360 | | | | | | 18 | 29.4 |
| *Professional, Business, Service* | −0.0941 | 0.0270 | | | | | | 84 | 31.8 |
| Landless Laborer | 0.3225 | 0.1700 | | | | | | 84 | 50.06 |

Grand Mean=2.16 Multiple $R^2$=0.2429 $F_1$=4.2718*

*Significant at the .05 level of confidence.

The unadjusted and adjusted coefficients basically indicate the deviations to the adjusted and unadjusted category means. The negative values indicate that the N.S. for particular category is better than the grand mean, whereas positive values indicate that the N.S. is lower than the grand mean. The adjusted coefficients, however, indicate the true effect of a predictor when others are held constant.

relationships. This is indicated by $F_2$, $F_3$ and $F_4$ tests in Table 6.1. Considering the strength of relationship and explanatory power in both bivariate and multivariate conditions, infection tendency and annual income of the family appear to be the most significant determinants. Since all the variables except quality of micro-environment have emerged significant in explaining in the N.S. behavior, each will be included in the discussion. In accordance with our earlier conceptualization in Chapter 4, each determinant is discussed under its identified domain.

## THE HEALTH DOMAIN

The infection tendency of the child and quality of living environment are discussed here in influencing the nutritional status of the child. Since infection tendency remained the most important predictor, it is discussed first.

### Infection Tendency of the Child and N.S.

In the present study the infection tendency of a child is ascertained and categorized as low, medium, or high on the basis of infection episodes told by the mother or grandmother in the occurrence of diarrhea (gastrointestinal infections), cough and cold (indicating upper and lower respiratory tract infections), and fever—generally of unknown origin.

The result of the MCA revealed infection tendency as the most closely associated variable with the N.S., even after adjusting the effect of other variables (see $eta^2$ and $beta^2$ values in Table 6.1). Obviously, it explained the maximum variation in the criterion variable. The gradient in the relationship of malnutrition with varying infection tendency is evident from the increasing coefficient values of the infection categories (Table 6.1). The results of prevalence analysis in Table 6.1 also indicate that children in the high infection category are more than twice as malnourished as their counterparts with low infections. Some possible causes for high infections leading to malnutrition are analyzed below.

According to our classification scheme more than two-thirds of the children observed had suffered from mild to severe infections. Occurrence of severe infections remained relatively

TABLE 6.2 : **Simple Correlation between Selected Variables Influencing the Nutritional Status**

| | Nutritional Status | Caste | Annual Income | Income Spent on Food | Infection Tendency | Quality of Micro Environment | Density of Rooms | Number of Children | Food Group of the Child | Sell Milk | Milk Consumption | Weaning | Age of Mother |
|---|---|---|---|---|---|---|---|---|---|---|---|---|---|
| Annual income of family | −0.240 | −0.120 | 1.00 | −0.616 | −0.120 | −0.424 | — | −0.150 | −0.188 | — | −0.377 | — | — |
| Infection Tendency | 0.278 | — | −0.120 | — | 1.000 | 0.199 | — | — | — | 0.194 | 0.125 | 0.152 | — |
| Quality of Micro-Environment | 0.240 | — | −0.424 | 0.348 | 0.199 | 1.000 | 0.183 | — | −0.148 | — | 0.243 | — | — |
| Number of Children | 0.216 | — | −0.150 | 0.136 | — | — | 0.195 | 1.000 | 0.123 | −0.124 | — | — | 0.66 |
| Food Group of the Child | −0.113 | 0.111 | 0.189 | — | — | −0.148 | — | −0.123 | 1.00 | — | — | — | — |
| Birth Interval | −0.180 | — | — | — | −0.119 | — | — | −0.298 | −0.187 | — | — | — | 0.40 |
| Occupation | 0.161 | 0.368 | −0.155 | — | — | 0.140 | — | — | −0.135 | — | 0.291 | — | — |
| Work Status of Mother | −0.123 | — | — | — | | 0.203 | — | — | — | — | — | 0.127 | — |

*(Contd.)*

TABLE 6.2 (*Contd.*)

| | Feeding practice | Food attitude | Hot-Cold food concept | Birth interval | Occupation | Work status of mother | Education of mother | Religion | Concept of Balanced diet | Family planning | Source of drinking water | Immunization status |
|---|---|---|---|---|---|---|---|---|---|---|---|---|
| Annual income of family | — | −0.262 | — | — | −0.155 | — | 0.337 | −0.174 | −0.153 | 0.121 | −0.191 | — |
| Infection Tendency | — | — | — | −0.119 | — | — | — | — | 0.155 | — | — | −0.223 |
| Quality of Micro-Environment | — | — | — | — | 0.141 | −0.203 | −0.344 | — | — | — | 0.174 | 0.189 |
| Number of Children | 0.145 | — | — | −0.299 | — | — | −0.212 | — | — | 0.352 | — | — |
| Food Group of the Child | — | — | — | −0.187 | −0.135 | — | 0.226 | — | −0.113 | — | — | — |
| Birth Interval | — | — | — | 1.000 | — | — | — | — | — | — | — | — |
| Occupation | −0.176 | 0.353 | 0.156 | — | 1.000 | 0.159 | −0.116 | 0.224 | — | — | — | — |
| Work Status of mother | −0.161 | 0.116 | — | — | 0.159 | 1.000 | 0.186 | — | 0.135 | — | 0.160 | — |

*Note*: Only those relationships significant at .05 level of significance are shown in the Table. Explanation for direction of relationships are given in the text.

TABLE 6.3 : **Simple Correlation[1] between Determinants of Mulnutrition and Nutritional Status of Children in the Sampled Villages**

| Village/ Predictor | Infection tendency | Quality of micro-environment | Family annual income | Birth interval | Number of children | Food group of the child | Work status of mother | Occupation of head of household |
|---|---|---|---|---|---|---|---|---|
| Manakpur | 0.576* | 0.447* | −0.541* | −0.002 | 0.403* | −0.024 | −0.421* | 0.324* |
| Mehra | −0.162 | −0.043 | −0.306 | 0.096 | 0.217 | −0.504* | −0.265 | 0.132 |
| Sangatpura | −0.252 | 0.332* | −0.507* | −0.047 | 0.430* | −0.298 | 0.024 | 0.086 |
| Salamkhera | −0.261 | 0.221 | −0.233 | −0.340* | −0.095 | −0.122 | −0.372* | 0.289 |
| Landheri | 0.244 | 0.289 | −0.114 | 0.184 | 0.343* | 0.181 | 0.173 | 0.034 |
| Chandi | 0.289 | 0.212 | 0.178 | 0.063 | 0.005 | −0.198 | −0.168 | 0.449* |
| Pirthala | 0.522* | 0.116 | −0.141 | 0.036 | 0.289 | 0.043 | 0.029 | 0.025 |
| Firozpur Namak | 0.301 | 0.393* | −0.324 | −0.007 | 0.382* | −0.106 | 0.124 | −0.110 |
| Sarangwas | 0.638* | 0.105 | −0.001 | −0.002 | 0.134 | −0.122 | 0.071 | 0.070 |
| Rajgarh | −0.164 | 0.445* | −0.518* | −0.332* | 0.328 | −0.102 | 0.231 | 0.080 |

*Correlation Coefficients significant at .05 confidence level.

[1]Spearman Rank Correlation Coefficients.

high among scheduled caste children, whereas low occurrence was noticed across the Khatri/Arora and Bishnoi children. Better personal hygiene and environmental sanitation among Khatri families most likely contributed to low infections. In general, infections remained high where environmental sanitation and personal hygiene were poor, children were closely spaced, income standards remained low, and weaning period started late (see Correlation Analysis Table 6.2). As a result of above conditions, the variable probably remained significantly related with N.S. in Manakpur, Pirthala. and Sarangwas villages (see Table 6.3). Infection episodes could have been lower if the children were immunized to most common childhood diseases. In the surveyed villages, more than 70 per cent of the children were not fully covered by available immunization programs. The full coverage was noticed only in village of Chandi where, under the auspices of the Integrated Child Development Scheme, extended medical and nutritional facilities were provided for the pre-school children. Under the domiciliary health services of the Haryana Health Department, the basic immunization program was also available in Firozpur Namak. Consequently, the infection tendencies in both villages were significantly low and so was the prevalence of malnutrition (Table 6.4).

How improved environmental sanitation and personal hygiene can lead to lower morbidity and thus better nutritional status can be illustrated from the following observation. Even without immunization facilities, the infectious episodes among young children of Sarangwas were observed to be among the lowest (Table 6.4). The reasons for low infections can be related to better environmental sanitation and personal hygiene habits introduced by the servicemen of this village. In comparison to most other villages, the quality of living conditions, as reflected in low density of rooms, absence of open drains, better location of animal rooms, and ventilation facilities, was much higher, more than 70 per cent of the heads of households (primarily Ahir caste) were reported either retired from or currently drafted in the military service. The Ahir dominant areas of southern Haryana remained the popular draft areas during the British *Raaj*. Most of these servicemen import improved sanitary and hygienic habits to their families. As a consequence of such

TABLE 6.4 : **Infection Episodes and Prevalence of PCM in the Studied Villages**

| Village | Low infection % | PCM III PCM IV % | Medium infection % | PCM III PCM IV % | High infection % | PCM III PCM IV % |
|---|---|---|---|---|---|---|
| Manakpur | 19.0 | 16.1 | 48.5 | 20.0 | 32.4 | 80.0 |
| Mehra | 19.4 | 57.1 | 33.3 | 33.0 | 47.3 | 29.1 |
| Sangatpura | 22.7 | 20.0 | 31.8 | 28.5 | 45.5 | 60.0 |
| Salamkhera | 37.1 | 23.0 | 22.9 | 50.0 | 40.0 | 57.0 |
| Landheri | 19.2 | 28.1 | 41.8 | 26.7 | 39.0 | 43.1 |
| Chandi | 43.2 | 18.1 | 32.4 | 25.0 | 24.4 | 66.6 |
| Pirthala | 26.4 | 14.0 | 34.6 | 33.3 | 38.8 | 60.1 |
| Firozpur Namak | 35.3 | 20.0 | 46.6 | 38.5 | 18.1 | 40.0 |
| Sarangwas | 51.5 | 7.0 | 25.9 | 28.6 | 22.6 | 83.3 |
| Rajgarh | 33.4 | 50.0 | 45.8 | 54.5 | 20.8 | 40.0 |
| Total Sample | 30.5 | 23.1 | 36.3 | 33.1 | 33.2 | 54.0 |

*Source*: Author's Field Work.

habits, it is likely that infection episodes were among the lowest in this village (Table 6.4) and the variable came out most significantly related with the N.S. (see Table 6.3). In contrast, the infection tendencies were noticed high in Manakpur children, particularly among the scheduled caste families. The quality of living conditions was very poor, except for the Khatri/Arora families. Both infection tendency and quality of living conditions probably contributed more to the poor N.S. of the sampled children of this village.

Among other possible causes of infection, water supply did not emerge significant as was expected. In the present study, except for Manakpur and Sangatpura where traditional dug wells are still the main source of drinking water, safe water was assured in other villages either by government operated piped water supply or privately installed hand pumps. It may be mentioned that despite the safe sources of drinking water, some families still prefer to use open well water for sanctity[3] or taste reasons. Since safe water was available to most children, the causation of infections related to water-borne bacteria is difficult to ascertain here. In summary, the influence of infection tendencies on the N.S. of the Haryana children seems strong. Such influence may be *indirectly* attributed to the poor quality of living conditions, close spacing of the children, inaccessibility to immunization programs, and late weaning. Most infected children were noticed in low income families, and generally belonged to the lower castes. The experience from a few villages suggests that if the immunization programs are within easy reach, and education in personal hygiene and sanitation is reinforced, high morbidity due to infections can be significantly reduced.

It may be cautioned at this point that due to the synergistic relationship between infection and malnutrition, it is also likely that malnutrition condition of a child itself contributes to infection tendency. Therefore, the results need to be interpreted with caution, since we cannot isolate this cyclical cause-effect relationship.

## ECONOMIC DOMAIN

Three aspects of the relationship between income and N.S. are addressed in this analysis. First, what is the statistical contribution of the income variable in explaining the variation in N.S. of the sampled children? Second, in what way does income influence the N.S.? Finally, and importantly, does increase in family income always insure a better N.S. for the children?

The income effect on the nutritional status was discussed briefly in the previous chapter, the prevalence of PCM III and PCM IV was observed to be more than three times greater in the low income group children than in their counterparts in the high income group (for comparison see Table 5.8). Evidently, its impact on the N.S. was strongly felt. At that time we did not examine the independent and spatial effect of this variable, rather, the emphasis remained on the prevalence pattern and identification of income/age related target groups. The former concern is discussed now.

The MCA analysis clearly revealed income as the second most important factor influencing variations in the N.S. across the entire sample (see beta square values in Table 6.1). Although the combined effect of other variables (possibly occupation and

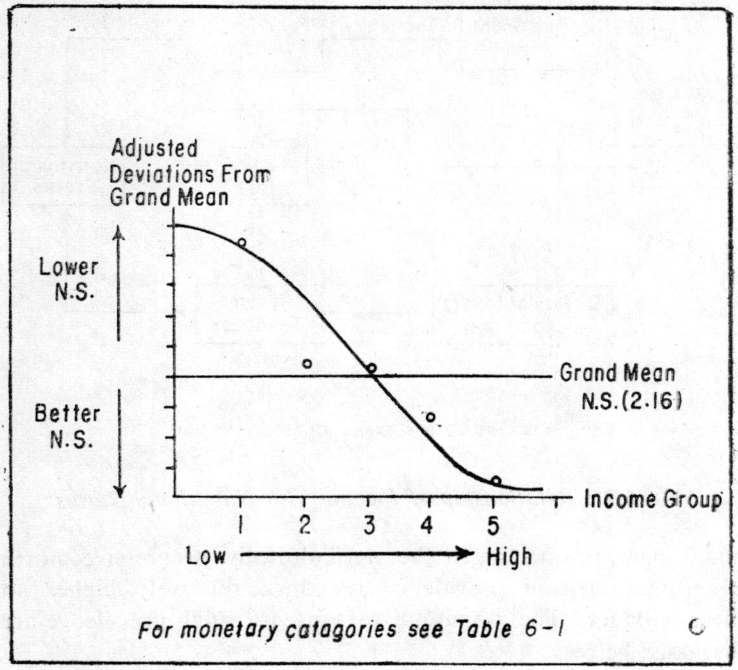


FIG. 6.1 : *Adjusted Deviations from the Grand Mean N.S. in Different Income Groups*

work status of mother) is visible from the lowered beta square values, its rank did not deflect even after holding constant the effects of other variables ($F_4$ test in Table 6.1). This indicates its strong individual influence on the N.S. The lowest and highest income group children deviated most from the adjusted grand mean (as evident from adjusted coefficients in Fig. 6.1 and Table 6.1). Children in other categories showed minuscule deviation. The high positive coefficient value for the Rs. 0-1200 group implies that children of the poorest families are highly malnourished. If income is the criterion of intervention, such families deserve first priority.

At the village level, income remained significantly related with N.S. in Manakpur and Sangatpura of the north zone, and Rajgarh of the south zone (Table 6.3). Although Manakpur

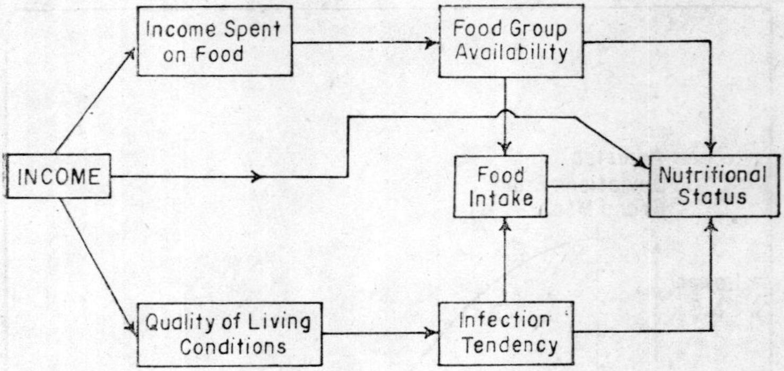


The arrows indicate significant relationship

FIG. 6.2 : *Relationship of Income with Nutritional Status*

and Sangatpura belong to the agriculturally progressive north zone, malnutrition prevalence remained relatively higher in these villages. The apparent reasons for high prevalence are discussed below.

Manakpur, located in the piedmont plain of Siwalik hills (see Fig. 4.2) and cut by seasonal streams, faces difficulties in implementation of agricultural development plans. Irrigation facilities are almost absent in the village (see Appendix A). Income levels were low for more than 50 per cent of the sample families except the business caste community of Ahluwalias. Not only food, but the quality of living conditions were degenerative as a result of very low incomes. High infection tendencies and large families further aggravated the income effect on the general health conditions. A similar, but less intense, situation was noticed in Sangatpura, located in the alluvial flood plain. Periodic flooding and low irrigation development kept the agricultural efficiency low for most small land holding families. Around two-thirds of the households in the sample subsisted on an income of less than Rs. 2400. Like Manakpur, low food availability and poor living conditions in the low income families most likely affected the N.S. of the young children. Rajgarh, situated in the undulating sandy tract of western Haryana, lacked most ingredients of economic development. Here, 75 per cent of the children belonged to low income group and more than two-thirds of them were observed to be malnourished.

In most other villages of the central and south zone, even with sand dune concentration and low rainfall reliability, development of canal irrigation, spurred by the political leadership of the area, helped in mitigating the low income effect on the N.S. Broadly stated, in villages which lacked agricultural development efforts, the poverty conditions generally aggravated the malnutrition problem.

**Influence of Income on the Nutritional Status**

As regards the second question, there seems to be indirect impact of income on N.S. through the intervening variables of food group and general health status (see Fig. 6.2). These two factors in return influence the N.S. The estimated relationships are shown in Fig. 6.2. In the present population we notice a significant correlation (Spearman Correlation Coefficient=0.188 $p>0.001$) between income of a family and the food group of the child.[4] Around 27 per cent of the children belonging to low income groups (income less than Rs. 2400) consumed carbohydrate dominant foods, whereas less than 3 per cent of the high income (income more than Rs. 8400) children subsisted on caloric dominant foods (Table 6.5). Likewise, out of 24 children who consumed a balanced diet in the entire sample, only two belonged to the low income group. That a large proportion of even rich families' children did not consume a balanced diet can be related to cultural factors or local unavailability of nutritious products such as vegetables and fruits. In the protein dominant group, variation due to income was not significant because most children in this group were young, and full or partial breast-feeding up to 18 months prevailed irrespective of economic status. Of course, N.S. in this group of children will vary with the post partum health conditions of the mother. Influence of living conditions on the infectious episodes has already been discussed in the previous section. As noted, the living conditions in rural Haryana are generally poor except for few social groups (Ahirs, Panjabis). Income influence further deteriorated the quality of living conditons, particularly in the low income families. Two-thirds of the sampled food families dwell

TABLE 6.5 : **Food Group Available in Different Income Group Children**

| Food group<br>Frequency<br>Per cent<br>ROW PCT<br>COL PCT | Income (Rs.) Below 1200 | 1201-2400 | 2401-4800 | 4801-8400 | Above 8400 | Total |
|---|---|---|---|---|---|---|
| | 15 | 43 | 28 | 20 | 16 | 122 |
| Protein Rich | 4.97 | 14.24 | 9.27 | 6.62 | 5.30 | 40.40 |
| | 12.30 | 35.25 | 22.95 | 16.39 | 13.11 | |
| | 44.12 | 43.00 | 37.84 | 38.46 | 38.10 | |
| | 13 | 23 | 7 | 7 | 1 | 51 |
| Carbohydrate | 4.30 | 7.62 | 2.32 | 2.32 | 0.33 | 16.89 |
| Rich | 25.49 | 45.10 | 13.73 | 13.73 | 1.96 | |
| | 38.24 | 23.00 | 9.46 | 13.46 | 2.38 | |
| | 6 | 32 | 32 | 19 | 16 | 105 |
| Protein and | 1.99 | 10.60 | 10.60 | 6.29 | 5.30 | 34.77 |
| Carbohydrate | 5.71 | 30.48 | 30.48 | 18.10 | 15.24 | |
| only | 17.65 | 32.00 | 43.24 | 36.54 | 38.10 | |
| | 0 | 2 | 7 | 6 | 9 | 24 |
| Balanced | 0.00 | 0.66 | 2.32 | 1.99 | 2.98 | 7.95 |
| | 0.00 | 8.33 | 29.17 | 25.00 | 37.50 | |
| | 0.00 | 2.00 | 9.46 | 11.54 | 21.43 | |
| Total | 34 | 100 | 74 | 52 | 42 | 302 |
| | 11.26 | 33.11 | 24.50 | 17.22 | 13.91 | 100.00 |

Kendall Tau B=0.16069 $p > 0.0009$
Spearman Correlation Coefficient=0.18847 $p > .0010$
*For categorization of food groups and inclusion of foods in each group please see Chapter 3.

in highly unsatisfactory conditions, compared to less than one-fourth of the rich families.

## Does Increase in Income Always Insure a Better N.S.?

The foregoing analysis demonstrated that nutritional status varied significantly with income. Can we conclude from such findings that the N.S. will rise in the poor families if their income is enchanced?

During the field enquiry the parents were asked about their expenditure behavior, if their income were to increase in future. Only one-third opted to spend on children's food. More than

TABLE 6.6 : **Expenditure Behavior with Increase in Income**

| Expenditure behavior<br>Frequency<br>Per cent<br>ROW PCT<br>COL PCT | Income (Rs.)<br>Below 1200 | 1201-2400 | 2401-4800 | 4801-8400 | Above 8400 | Total |
|---|---|---|---|---|---|---|
| Child (Food) | 10<br>3.31<br>9.80<br>29.41 | 37<br>12.25<br>36.27<br>37.00 | 26<br>8.61<br>25.49<br>35.14 | 18<br>5.96<br>17.65<br>34.62 | 11<br>3.64<br>10.78<br>26.19 | 102<br>33.77 |
| Social | 20<br>6.62<br>12.82<br>58.82 | 47<br>15.56<br>30.13<br>47.00 | 39<br>12.91<br>25.00<br>52.70 | 23<br>7.62<br>14.74<br>44.23 | 27<br>8.94<br>17.31<br>64.29 | 156<br>51.66 |
| Child and Social | 4<br>1.32<br>9.09<br>11.76 | 16<br>5.30<br>36.36<br>16.00 | 9<br>2.98<br>20.45<br>12.16 | 11<br>3.64<br>25.00<br>21.15 | 4<br>1.32<br>9.09<br>9.52 | 44<br>14.57 |
| Total | 34<br>11.26 | 100<br>33.11 | 4<br>24.50 | 52<br>17.22 | 42<br>13.91 | 302<br>100.00 |

Kendall Tau B=0.0207 p $\geqslant$ 0.6775

Spearman Correlation Coefficient=0.02425 p $\geqslant$ 0.6747

half proposed to spend on social purposes, and less than 15 per cent for both purposes (Table 6.6). In low income families (less than Rs. 2400) only 35 per cent indicated additional expenditure on children with future rise of income. Increase in income in the poor countries may not always ensure a proportionate expenditure on food. Except in very poor families whose children are not meeting basal physiological food needs, it is more likely that additional income may be disbursed elsewhere—payment of debt, marriage, house, agricultural implements, etc. As evident from the present analysis, cultural, social or familial norms seem so forceful that additional income does not imply a better quality of food, and hence an improved nutritional status. Apparently, unless the social needs of the low income families are met, a small increase in income may have little impact in improving N.S. through expenditure on food.

The above findings indicate that although N.S. varies with income in a general sense, it is not realistic to conclude that an increase in income will ensure better health for all income groups due to increased expenditure on food. The relationship of N.S. with income is probably significant for very poor and very rich populations. If we look back at Table 6.1, we find that the adjusted mean in the income range of Rs. 1201 to Rs. 8400 is not significantly different from the grand mean, whereas it is significantly different for the lowest and highest income groups. Evidently, children living in very poor families are the most critical group needing food and other intervention programs.

## DEMOGRAPHIC DOMAIN

The hypothesized relationship of some components of this domain with the N.S. has been detailed in Chapter 4. We mentioned at that point that the intervening variables most influencing N.S. seem to be spacing between births and the family size (considered in terms of number of children). Now we shall examine their statistical relationship with the N.S. in the sampled population as a whole, and across different villages of the study area.

### Impact of Birth Interval on the N.S.

Birth interval was determined by taking the age difference of the last two born children and is categorized at an 18 months interval. Those families having only one child are considered toward high spacing and are included in a separate category to examine their distinct effect.

Birth interval came out as the fourth most significant variable in the classification analysis, and was negatively related to the N.S. (see Table 6.1). A negative relationship indicates that the nutritional status worsens as the spacing between the last two consecutive children is reduced. This was expected according to our conceptualization (see Chapter 3). The relatively higher rank of this variable in a multivariate situation suggests that spacing alone does not explain as much variation as it does when considered with other variables. Possibly its negative relationship with family size enhanced its explanatory power. The

TABLE 6.7 : **Comparison of Hyderabad and Haryana Children in Relation to Spacing between Births and Prevalence of Malnutrition**

| Hyderabad Study* | | Haryana Study | |
|---|---|---|---|
| Inter-pregnancy interval (months) | Per cent malnourished children | Spacing between births (months) | Per cent malnourished children (PCM III and PCM IV)** |
| Less than 12 | 56.2 | Less than 18 | 38.9 |
| 12-23 | 62.3 | 19-36 | 42.7 |
| 24-35 | 56.3 | 37 and above | 26.3 |
| 36-47 | 37.8 | only child | 28.3 |
| 48 and above | 28.6 | | |

**Source*: Agit Kumar *et al.*, "Study of Morbidity in Pre-school Children of Rural Hyderabad in Relation to Family Size and Birth Interval," *Indian Pediatrics* 12 (1976), 123-26.

**For explanation of PCM categories see Chapter 4.

category effect as set out in Table 6.1 indicates that about two-thirds of the children were born at an interval of 36 months or below, and about 40 per cent of them were malnourished. As the interval increased to more than 36 months the malnutrition rate dropped to 26 per cent. As expected, malnourished remained low in the only child category. The beta value and adjusted coefficients for the categories reinforced our findings that even after considering the effect of other variables, N.S. remained significantly higher for less closely spaced children.

Our results correspond greatly to another study conducted for pre-school children of rural Hyderabad. The results of both studies are compared in Table 6.7. From both studies it is apparent that malnourishment among young children declines abruptly if the children are spaced at a more than three-year interval.

Now we look for the reasons that possibly account for lower nutritional status in closely spaced children. In general, children with a low birth interval had a higher incidence of infections that may contribute to their lower N.S. Since natural immunization available from human milk gets reduced in closely spaced children, the aggravation of infections while living in poor environmental conditions seems imminent.

Furthermore, a cursory examination of spacing and nutritional status was also utilized through surrogates such as age of the mother, size of the family, and adoption of modern family planning methods. The age of the mother came out as the most significantly related surrogate with birth interval (Table 6.2). Young mothers tended to have closely spaced children, whereas average birth gap increased in children born to older mothers. In the case of rural Haryana, marriages at an early age (ranging from 15 to 19 years for girls) are common, and due to minuscule adoption of family planning methods, fertility is usually greater. In the present study, mothers below 35 years of age constituted 86 per cent of sample and 78 per cent of them (or their husbands) never used any modern family planning methods. Spacing between births was closest among such mothers. In addition, families of large size and with few family planning practices were also noticed to have closely spaced children (Table 6.2). In brief, it is inferred from the above relationships that if the young mothers space their children close to the three-year interval, the low possibility of infections and better health care may lead to improve nutritional status of their children.

**Impact of Family Size on the N.S.**

The family size was determined by counting the number of live children in the sampled family. A small size family is considered to have two or fewer children, whereas a large size family is viewed to include more than four children. It was believed in our conceptualization (Chapter 3) that large size families might have a higher prevalence of malnutrition principally due to low per caput availability of food and poor quality of living conditions, such as crowding.

The above relationships are found to be true according to our correlation analysis and MCA results (see Tables 6.1 and 6.2). The prevalence figures in Table 6.1 clearly point to the fact that the prevalence of PCM remained almost two times higher in large size families as compared to those included in the small size family category. In a more rigorous manner the MCA model confirmed that family size is a significant explanator of N.S. either independently or along with the effect of other associated variables (see $eta^2$ and $beta^2$ values in Table 6.1). The precise behavior of N.S. with varying family size is also explicit from the adjusted and unadjusted coefficients' variation in the three family size categories. The drop in adjusted coefficients for the small size family (two or less children) suggests the multicollinearity effect of other variables. It is more likely that this category contained more of the healthier young children belonging to the protein group (fully breast-fed) and only child categories. In other categories such influences seem negligible, as the adjusted and unadjusted coefficients fluctuate little. Evidently, the small size family children were significantly better nourished.

While looking for the association of family size with other variables which indirectly influence the N.S., birth interval, education of mother, family planning, density of rooms, income, selling of milk, and food group of the child emerged as possible surrogates (see correlation Table 6.2). The major influence of family size was noticed in the availability of food group to a child. Most children in large families subsisted on tea and carbohydrate foods. The unavailability of milk in some large Jat and Ahir families of Chandi, Rajgarh, and Sarangwas was reported due to the milk selling practice. Although the selling of milk is not common among Jats, economic necessity due to large family size and proximity to a major urban center (such as Rohtak, Bhiwani, Rewari) prompted them to engage in this practice. Nutritionally, young children suffered more as milk got replaced with tea in the diet pattern. The large family size also affected the general health conditions by creating poor quality living conditions. Crowding remained relatively high in such families, as one bedroom was shared by more than five persons in at least 75 per cent of the families. The probability of spreading droplet infections is greatly enhanced in closely spaced children under crowded conditions. Briefly, the high infection tendency of and low food availability to sampled children born in large size families probably contributed to their lower N.S. Such influences were noticed to be strong in Meo and Jat families.

For the demographic domain, in general, it is concluded that children in large size families, usually with a short birth interval, show lower nutritional status. Little practice of family planning results in large size families and closely spaced children. Low food availability and poor quality of living conditions generally lead to higher infections and lower nutritional status in most such families. The spatial importance of this domain is realized by the fact that the demographic variables remained strongly correlated in all the three zones (see Table 6.3) and particularly within the villages of Manakpur and Sangatpura of the north zone, Salamkhera and Landheri of the central zone, and Firozpur Namak and Rajgarh of the south zone. The findings in this section reinforce our earlier view in Chapter 3 (Demographic Domain) that population and health problems in a community should be addressed together, if the relationships between the two problems are found convincing.

## DIETARY DOMAIN

It may be recalled from the previous discussion on conceptualization that food intake of a child was classified into four major food groups: (*i*) protein dominant, (*ii*) carbohydrate dominant, (*iii*) mixed (mixture of group (*i*) and group (*ii*), and (*iv*) balanced (group (*iii*), and vegetables, fruits, and lipids). It was hypothesized that the dietary domain should come out a very significant explanator due to its direct relationship to N.S. through metabolism. It is also expected that mixed and balanced food groups might contain healthier children due to their occurrence in rich, small size, and educated families who can afford and are possibly aware of the nutrition concept. In spatial terms, little significant variation is expected in food group behavior across villages because the sample contains young children and their food intake is not much influenced by agricultural potential or cropping patterns of different villages, rather, it is influenced indirectly by micro-environment and economic, social, cultural or demographic peculiarities. However, a general spatial analysis will be presented to show how agricultural revolution and urbanization forces could influence the food pattern and availability of certain nutritious food groups in different ecological settings.

In the classification analysis the food group of the child came out as a significant explanator in both bivariate and multivariate relationships (see Table 6.1). The lowered variance in the multivariate situation is possibly due to its indirect relationship to economic and demographic variables. Moreover, its lower rank in the hierarchy of predictors might have been influenced by the overlapping nature of food categories. For a detailed understanding of this domain, the categorical analysis with prevalence pattern of PCM is illustrated below.

### Protein Rich Food Group

This group contained around 40 per cent of the sampled children and their diets consisted primarily of human and animal milk, milk products (yogurt, buttermilk) or a variety of pulses (legumes). Human milk remained the most important protein food due to the age factor. Eighty-five per cent of the children in this group were below 18 months and 75 per cent of them were partially or fully breast-fed. Meat and animal milk constituted another major protein food for a few older children belonging to the Meo and Bishnoi castes respectively.[5] Pulses did not dominate *per se*. However, in combination with other cereals they provided major protein supply in a few cultivator caste families. The prevalence of PCM remained moderate in this group (see Fig. 6.3). The major sufferers were those older children who subsisted on partial breast-feeding and received an inadequate amount of calories from scant supplementary foods. These children can be counted toward a kwashirkor syndrome.

The negligible difference in the adjusted and unadjusted coefficients signifies little influence of exogenous variables on the children in this food group. Probably the common breast-feeding practice among most economic, social, and cultural groups kept the varying influence of such factors low.

### Carbohydrate Rich Food Groups

Fifty-one children belonged to this group and 61 per cent of them came out malnourished (see Fig. 6.3). A large majority of children in this cluster were older and belonged to low income families and within scheduled castes. As the children entered the early weaning stage, especially due to close spacing of the next child, probably their enhanced food needs could not be served by carbohydrate rich cereals (wheat, rice, corn, barley and millets) and jaggery alone. Deficiency of proteins, minerals,

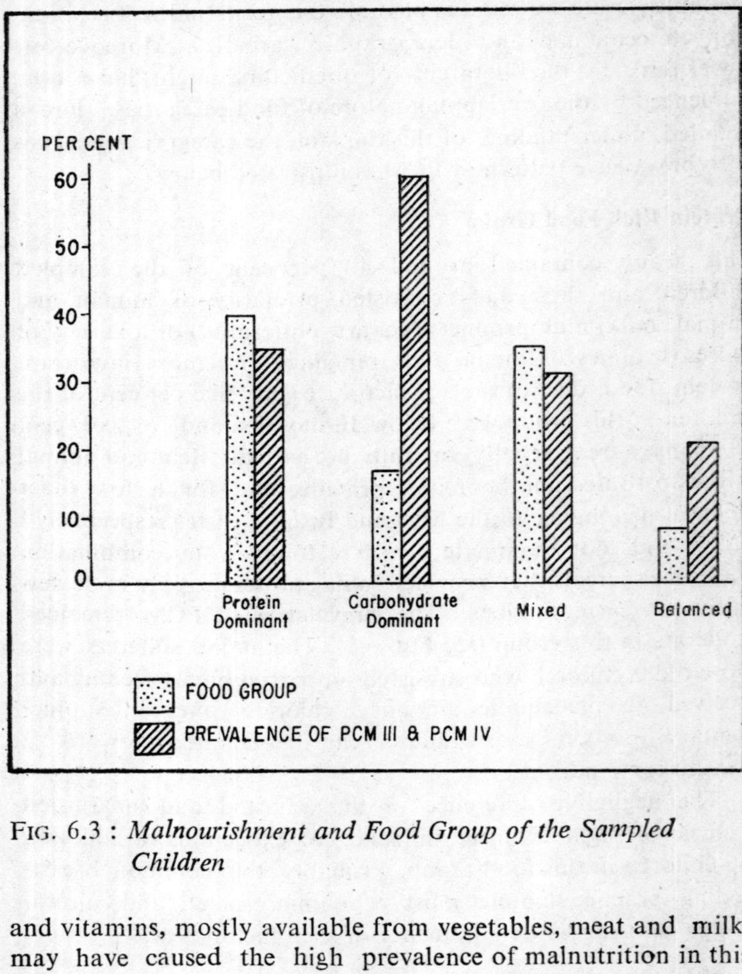


FIG. 6.3 : *Malnourishment and Food Group of the Sampled Children*

and vitamins, mostly available from vegetables, meat and milk, may have caused the high prevalence of malnutrition in this group.

From the category analysis we find that even after holding constant the effect of other variables, the adjusted coefficients still showed a maximum deviation from the grand mean. Obviously, the exogenous variables such as income and family size lowered the malnourishment rate (as reflected in lowered coefficients in Table 6.1). However, unless a variety of foods are added in the diet pattern, the nutrition problem cannot be solved completely in this food group children.

## Mixed and Balanced Food Groups

As expected, a relatively small proportion of children emerged malnourished in these groups (Fig. 6.3). We are not certain whether most subjects were receiving the recommended allowance of nutrients, nevertheless, probably, the variety in food helped in providing the essential nutrients which kept the malnutrition rate substantially low, at least in the balanced food group children.

The categorical analysis reveals that children in the mixed groups remained close to the grand mean and other variables had little influence in changing the N.S. Since most children in this food group have crossed the crucial weaning stage, and the availabilities of carbohydrate and protein rich foods in the form of *chapattis* (unleavened bread), parboiled rice, *dahl* (protein rich thick soup of lentiles and pulses), and miscellaneous local snacks (baked and green chikpea, popcorn) and drinks (sugarcane juice) essentially kept the malnutrition rate moderately low across all socio-economic groups.

Surprisingly, due to the inclusion of vegetables, fruits, and some lipids in the 'balanced' food groups, the malnutrition prevalence declined to almost 20 per cent (Fig. 6.3). At the same time the possible influence of other variables such as income and family size became strong in this category of children as revealed by the lowered adjusted coefficients in Table 6.1. It was found that children included in the balanced diet group belonged to small size families and high income groups. When the influence of these and other variables is held constant, the coefficients decline, indicating their positive influence on the balanced food group children.

Evidently, only a small proportion of the sample including very rich and/or small size families could afford expensive diets containing fruits, vegetables, and animal or vegetable fats. Nearly 90 per cent subsisted on relatively poor to moderate food groups. Income, occupation, size of the family, spacing, education of the mother, and caste came out as possible reasons for belonging to a balanced or poor food group (see correlation analysis: Table 6.2). Except caste, the specific relationship of other influencing variables has already been discussed in the previous sections.

Indirectly, urbanization and cropping patterns in different areas of Haryana were also felt to be important surrogates in affecting the availability or choice of different food groups. Their possible relationship with food groups is discussed below.

**Urbanization Impact on Food Group**

Rapid growth of large cities and closely spaced urban centers have created a lucrative demand for milk. Favored sites of milk demand are along the major highways, and surrounding the urban centers. Among our studied villages, around 40 per cent families in Chandi, Sarangwas and Rajgarh sold milk to their nearest urban centers. Surprisingly, milk selling was getting popular even among those castes (such as Jats and Ahirs) who once considered this practice against their religious beliefs or as social stigma to their prestige. Unfortunately, as a result of this practice, tea has been ingrained in the diet pattern of adults as well as young children across most villages. Leaving aside the very young breast-fed children, tea was consumed by more than 90 per cent of children over 2 years old as a full or partial substitute for milk. Although the popularity of tea and low consumption of milk is ascribed here to urbanization forces, most households attributed its relationship to economic factors, modernization syndrome, and medicinal qualities (particularly for the common cold and cough). In order to understand the precise relationship of the urbanization forces and protein deficiency, further research is suggested on the older children and adults around the major urban centers.

**The Green Revolution Impact**

A variety of legumes such as chick peas (*Cicer arietinum*), *urad* (*Phaseolus radiatus*), *moong* (*Phaseolus aureus*), *arhar* (*Cajanus cajan* or pigeon pea), and *masur* (*Lens esulentus* or *lentils*) along with *chapatti* (unleavened pancakes made of regional grains) dominate the diet pattern of most adults and older children in rural Haryana. Of all the *dahls* (soupy type preparation of the legumes), chick peas dominate in consumption due to their extensive production and variety of uses. It will be no exaggeration to say that in Haryana, *dahls* provide the principal share of protein requirements for adults as well as children.

However, under the impact of Green Revolution the low yielding legumes are facing tough competition from high yielding foodgrains (rice, wheat, corn), and other commercial crops (mainly sugarcane and cotton). Singh has clearly portrayed such a declining trend in the legumes acreage in his Agricultural Atlas of Haryana.[6] According to his findings, the per cent of total harvested area under chick peas (the principal legume) and other pulses has declined from almost 34 per cent, before the Green Revolution, to almost 18 per cent during 1970-73.[7] In eastern Haryana, acreage in mixed cropping of wheat and gram (a variety of chick peas) has almost dropped one-third due to the single cropping practice of wheat alone.[8] The cultivation of pulses is getting pushed to the marginal lands where water is at a premium and the soils are of poor quality. Even within the chick peas dominant areas of western and southern Haryana, high yielding variety foodgrains and commercial crops are making inroads with the diffusion of the inputs of Green Revolution.

By comparing the cropping pattern across the studied villages (see Appendix A), we also notice an inverse relationship between irrigation (one of the most important ingredients of the Green Revolution), and per cent of cultivated area under pulses. Mehra, a typical "Green Revolution" village, has only about 6 per cent area under pulses. Contrastingly, the poorly irrigated villages of Rajgarh and Firozpur Namak with sandy-clay soils devote more than 40 per cent of their cultivated area to pulses. Incidently, the malnutrition prevalence is among the lowest in Firozpur Namak (see Table 5.4). In other semi-arid villages (such as Landheri and Chandi) acreage under pulses is shrinking as irrigation facilities increase. The nutritional consequences of such a trend can be significant in future, although they are less perceptible now.

Furthermore, the earlier mentioned deficiencies in vegetables and fruits may be ascribed to a variety of factors. Haryana cultivators, in general, were observed to be less enthusiastic about truck farming or even kitchen gardening operations, except in areas very close to the urban centers. Lack of marketing facilities, increasing competition from the high yielding varieties of foodgrains, need for intensive care, and local pilfering by the non-growers usually discouraged cultivators from growing produce or seasonal fruits, in spite of the lucrative demand from the expanding urban centers. For example, mango, once the most popular seasonal fruit of Haryana, is becoming less available due to the clearing of mango groves for farming purposes. Other fruits (such as bananas, apples, grapes, etc.) are not grown locally due to climatic factors and are beyond the reach of most poor families. In the present sample, vegetable and fruit consumption remained relatively higher in villages located close to the urban centers (*viz.*, Manakpur, Mehra, Chandi, Pirthala), whereas in less favourably located villages the consumption remained satisfactory only in a few rich families.

## SOCIAL AND CULTURAL DOMAIN

The indirect influence of socio-cultural factors on the N.S. is usually subsumed under economic, demographic, health, and food group domains. Most such influences have already been discussed in the preceding analyses. At this point only those variables are examined which have direct bearing on the N.S. and were not emphasized earlier.

### SOCIAL FACTORS

Social impact is analyzed in relation to work status of the mother and occupation of the head of household. These two variables are discussed in detail as they emerge significant explanators in the classification analysis (Table 6.1).

#### Work Status of the Mother

In the present study, about 46 per cent of the mothers were observed to be engaged in farming operations either as helpmate to their husbands or to supplement the family's income. As expected, a large proportion of them belonged to farming castes of Hindu Jats and Ahirs. By tradition, most Hindu Jat and Ahir women of the central and south zones participate in most farming operations, except plowing. In contrast, within farming communities of north Haryana, full time participation of women in farm operations is culturally less acceptable except during the peak seasons, and then only for minor jobs. Female participation is also observed to be strong within Harijan and Balmiki castes (major scheduled castes) primarily for economic reasons. These castes are distributed all over Haryana and their participation in the work-force remained high in all villages. To what extent the work status of the mother influenced the N.S. of a child is apparent from the prevalence analysis and MCA results (see Table 6.1). According to the prevalence pattern, 45 per cent of the children of working mothers were noticed to be malnourished, compared to 30 per cent among non-working mothers' children. The statistical significance of this variable is apparent from the MCA results as the lower values for adjusted and unadjusted coefficients signify better nutritional standards for those children whose mothers are not engaged in full-time work. What possible factors or reasons are responsible for lower nutritional status of young children in working families is our next concern.

The correlation analysis in Table 6.2 demonstrates the fact that most working mothers belonged to small or medium size cultivating families, and their educational standards were relatively low. Furthermore, the working mothers most likely influenced the N.S. of their children due to early weaning practices without adequate supplementation. This was particularly evident among scheduled caste families. Natural immunization available through prolonged breast-feeding made a limited impact in containing infections among young children belonging to working mothers. Only 30 per cent of the working mothers could continue breast-feeding beyond nine months, while non-working mothers fed their siblings, on the average, for 18 months. The protein supply and natural immunization were thus inhibited to some extent among the working mothers' children. Poor quality of living, especially among the scheduled caste children, further aggravated the infection-malnutrition synergism.

**Occupation of the Head of Household**

Occupation came out as the third most important predictor, in spite of its strong relationship with other variables (particularly income). Its emergence as a significant explanator is probably due to its strong relation with caste (see Table 6.2), which has not been included in the model. In other words, occupation in the rural Haryana context can be considered a proxy variable of caste. Most Jat, Ahir, and Bishnoi were observed as small to big cultivators, whereas scheduled and artizan castes formed the largest labor group. Brahmin, Vaishya and Arora, were mostly engaged in the business or professional service activities.

In the category analysis (Table 6.1), we noticed that children belonging to the landless laborers (mostly low income) were the most malnourished, even after adjusting the influence of other factors. It was postulated that children belonging to professional business, and large cultivator families would show better nutrition status due to higher income and education factor. The positive adjusted coefficients for these categories indicate that when the influence of other factors in the model is held constant, the nutritional status of the children gets lower. It shows that higher N.S. in this category is principally due to some of the included variables in the model. The same reasoning appears to be true for large and medium cultivating families. On the contrary, the N.S. of children in small cultivating families gets better when the effect of factors such as income, family size, and quality of living conditions are adjusted. This influence is apparent from the lower negative adjusted coefficients as compared to higher unadjusted coefficients when such influences are not adjusted. Apparently, the N.S. in small cultivating and landless laborers' children can be significantly higher if the quality of living conditions, food availability, and income levels are raised. Concurrently, the rich occupational groups need to improve their food habits to keep up the health standards of their children with the existing income standards. Since occupation is significantly related to caste, specific influences of extraneous factors on the varying nutritional status across occupational groups will be discussed in the following caste analysis.

## CULTURAL FACTORS

Among important cultural factors influencing N.S., caste usually is considered the most important cultural variables in Indian context. This is due to its overriding influence on decisions about food choices, food preparation, and practices related to child weaning and feeding. The importance of this variable as an important surrogate of malnutrition was realized in Chapter 5 where prevalence of PCM differed significantly across various major castes (see Table 5.11). Children belonging to scheduled, artizan and Brahmin/Vaishya castes were observed to be most malnourished, whereas more healthly children were noticed across Jat Sikh, Bishnoi, and Khatri/Arora castes. At that time an investigation of the malnutrition problem across different caste children was not done. That concern is focused on now.

In analyzing the determinants of malnutrition, caste was not included in the MCA model due to its possible confounded relationship with several primary or secondary factors of malnutrition. Later, this was noticed true for at least occupation, income, and food group variables (see correlation Table 6.2). At this point, influence of caste on N.S. is analyzed in a more descriptive way through selected dietary variables which have direct bearing on the food intake of the child. These variables include feeding and weaning practices, food attitude and belief in hot and cold foods.

## Feeding Practices Among Major Castes

Full to partial breast-feeding remained popular in more than two-thirds of the families. Within major castes, breast-feeding was most common among scheduled castes, artizans, and farming Jat families. The practice also remained customary among non-working mothers and small size families. Poverty was among the limiting factors for most scheduled and artizan castes in choosing breast-feeding for longer time. For Jat mothers it was almost a traditional belief to breast-feed their children for better health. Directions of the elderly, especially the grandmother, were decisive in the practice of breast-feeding of babies by young mothers.

Lactation was generally prolonged. The period varied from six months to three years. Prolonged breast-feeding was more common among Jat and scheduled castes. The working mothers in Jat and scheduled caste families generally used the breast-feeding practice as a reward to their children after returning from work, even though the milk supply may be inadequate to meet any nutritional requirement or to satisfy hunger.

Breast-feeding is so deeply rooted in the cultural heritage that suckling is not considered merely as ingestion of food, but as a link or continuity between the mother and the child. Bottle-feeding is usually considered a last resort and scheduled feeding is taken by most as irrelevant.

Bottle-feeding was noticed more commonly among Meo, Bishnoi, Ahir, and Khatri/Arora castes. Modernization influences in keeping up the shape of the body was the perceived reasoning among the Khatri, Vaishya, Ahir and Bishnoi mothers.

In general, the breast-fed children were found to be better nourished irrespective of income or social status of the family. The practice remained common in all studied villages.

## Weaning Practices Among Major Castes

In the present study early weaning (at 6 months) were common among Jat/Sikh and Bishnoi families, whereas late weaning (after 12 months) was reported by Brahmin/Vaishya and Meo families. Farming communities of Jats and Ahirs, along with scheduled castes, were least particular about age of weaning, whereas business castes generally believed that weaning should start after one year. Possibly due to this belief, Brahmin/Vaishya caste children were more malnourished although their incomes were relatively high. Due to female participation in the work-force, early weaning was common among Jats, Ahirs, and scheduled castes' families also.

The cultural, economic, and spatial influences were more pronounced in selection and preparation of weaning foods. Carbohydrate rich weaning foods were common among the poor families, and protein or mineral rich foods dominated within very rich families. Type of weaning foods varied from area to area. *Khichri* (a mixture of cooked rice, moong pulse, with little *ghee*) was typical in north Haryana families, whereas *Dalia* (a paste of wheat/bajra flour with sugar syrup and *ghee*) is customary in south zone villages. Except in a few rich families, little preference was given to fruits and vegetables. When asked about giving green vegetables to the infants, most of the mothers were surprised to know that such things could ever be given to a baby.

**Belief in Hot and Cold Foods and the N.S.**

The concept of hot and cold food encourages or discourages consumption of some foods during specific seasons due to their culturally anticipated 'hot' or 'cold' effect on the brain or body in general. This is more entrenched in communities who believe in an Ayurvedic medicine system.[9] The nutritional implications are obvious in this belief as some nutritious foods (see Table 6.8) are abstained from irrespective of their nutritional value. The observance of this pseudo belief was felt to be strong among the non-farming Khatri/Arora and Brahmin/Vaishya communities. Other castes (particularly farming castes) also prohibited use of some nutritious foods, but were unconscious of the hot and cold food concept.

Although no significant correlation was observed between this concept and N.S. of the child, the concept does indicate a bearing on the N.S. in those families (particularly Brahmin and Vaishya) where such avoidances may be more rigidly observed.

In brief, the influence of cultural variables on the N.S. of a child was hard to measure. Their indirect influence on the N.S. could be considerable through food practices such as weaning, feeding, belief in hot and cold foods, and other food attitudes.

**Conclusions**

The following conclusions can be reached from the preceding analysis:

*Health Domain*

The infection tendency of the child remained the most significant explanator of malnutrition. Episodes of infection remained high even in rich families, suggesting that unless environmental sanitation is improved, income alone is not going to help in ameliorating malnutrition. Only in those villages where immunization programs were operative infection episodes remained low. This suggests the utility of the immunization programs in reducing infections and supports planned efforts to cover all children with basic immunization. In addition, infections were also high in families where children were closely spaced, and the weaning period started late. Also, the synergism between malnutrition and infections cannot be overlooked in attributing infection as the leading cause of malnutrition.

TABLE 6.8: **'Hot' and 'Cold' Foods Prohibited to the Children in the Haryana Study**

| Hot Foods in Summer | Cold Foods in Winter |
|---|---|
| *Meat and Poultry* | *Milk Products* |
| Egg | Yogurt |
| Meat | Butter milk |
| Fish | Skimmed milk |
| | Butter |
| *Vegetables and Fruits* | *Fruits and Juice* |
| Potato | Orange (orange juice) |
| Eggplant | Apple |
| Onion | Sugarcane juice |
| Methi (Fenugreek leaves) | |
| Mango | |
| *Pulses and Legumes* | *Vegetables* |
| Lentils | Reddish |
| Chick peas | Spinach |
| Kidney beans | Gourds |
| Arhar (Cajanus Cajan) | |
| *Beverages* | *Cereals* |
| Coffee | Wheat |
| Tea | Rice |
| | Barley |
| *Others* | |
| Spices | |
| Western Medicines | |

*Source*: Author's Field Wcrk.

## Income Domain

Most malnourished children were observed in the poorest families. The children in this category need planned intervention to correct malnutrition. In spatial terms, in the villages where agricultural development efforts lacked, the poverty conditions generally aggravated the malnutrition problem. Income influence was least on the young children, as most of them were breast-fed. After 12 months age, the income effect aggravates the malnutrition problem in low income families. The 'perceived' expenditure behavior with increase in income in the poor families revealed that social needs take priority over health. Small increases in income supposedly have little influence in enhancing the health status, unless some supplementary aid in terms of food or subsidized better housing is provided to improve the quality of life.

*Demographic Domain*

Less closely spaced children and those belonging to small size families were better nourished due to food availability and natural immunization available through breast-feeding. The study noticed that if the children are spaced close to a 3-year interval, the malnourishment declines abruptly.

*Dietary Domain*

Protein rich foods remained dominant among younger children, whereas carbohydrates provided most food needs of the older children. The latter was typically true in low income families of small cultivators and scheduled castes. In this study we notice that carbohydrates (major source of calories) are no major problem, whereas some deficiency is noticed for protein rich foods due to increasing urbanization and Green Revolution influences. Cultivable areas for major legumes were on a decline and the families located close to major urban centers were engaged in milk selling activities. Both practices affected the protein supply. The true estimates of protein deficiency cannot be stated here, since no diagnostic food consumption analysis was preformed. Quality food, rich in protein, minerals, and vitamins, was rare except in a few rich families at each location. The villages located in physically problematic areas such as Manakpur, Rajgarh and Firozpur Namak, faced more food availability problem, at least in the low income families.

*Socio-Cultural Domain*

Children of working mothers are more malnourished than those who do not actively participate in the farming operation. Hindu Jat and scheduled caste families had most of such children. The influence of caste was not estimated through MCA analysis; however, a descriptive analysis did indicate that children belonging to scheduled and artizan castes were the least nourished. Abject poverty was the major deterrent in availability of nutritious foods. Poor environmental conditions further triggered the malnourishment syndrome. The synergism between poverty, infection, and malnutrition was best

TABLE 6.9 : **Target Groups and Villages Based on Predictors**

| Predictor | Rank | Children in Critical Category needing Interventions (Based on MCA Results) | Villages where the Predictors remained significantly related with N.S. (Based on Correlation Analysis) |
|---|---|---|---|
| Infection | 1 | Children with very high infection tendency | Manakpur, Pirthala, Sarangwas |
| Income | 2 | Children of very low income families | Manakpur, Mehra, Sangatpura, Firozpur Namak, Rajgarh |
| Occupation | 3 | Children belonging to small cultivators and landless laborers | Manakpur, Chandi |
| Birth Interval | 4 | Children born within 18 months of each other | Salamkhera, Rajgarh |
| Work Status of Mother | 5 | Children of Working Mothers | Manakpur, Salamkhera |
| Food Group | 6 | Children Subsisting on Carbohydrate foods | Mehra |
| Number of Children | 7 | Children belonging to families with five and more children | Manakpur, Sangatpura, Landheri, Firozpur Namak |

explicable in this group of children. To effectuate any policy towards better health a tripartite approach involving family planning, health planning, and economic development seems more practical than a piecemeal strategy. The high prevalence of malnutrition within the Bania/Brahmin castes reflects that income is not the only inhibiting factor; rather, poor food habits such as late weaning, bottle-feeding, and a strong belief in hot and cold foods may be responsible factors for lower nutritional status.

Based on correlation coefficients for each predictor, the target groups shown in Table 6.9 are identified for the studied population. For orchestrating any intervention programs depending on the objectives, such groups can be considered the potential respondents for correcting the malnutrition problem. The limitation of the above analysis, however, must be understood. The villages in the study may not represent all the zonal characteristics because of the small number selected from each zone. Nevertheless, the 'target groups' noted above can be identified from each relationship with the nutritional status.

## REFERENCES

1. The independent variables are those possible determinants of N.S. which were identified in Table 3.3 of conceptualization chapter.
2. Andrews *et al.*, *Multiple Classification Analysis*, pp. 33-44.
3. The hand pumps use a *leather* washer. This fact makes the hand pump water impure for some religious people, who are pure vegetarians. Like myriad objects of worship in Indian mythology, the well is also worshipped in rural Haryana as a deity—source of lifegiving water. Some die-hard families for sanctity reasons prefer to use well water even though the hand pump is installed at home.
4. A detailed discussion on the relation of food groups with N.S. and other variables is given in a later section of this chapter.
5. Within Bishnoi caste, no meal is considered complete if it does not include milk products such as yogurt, buttermilk, and particularly *ghee* (clarified butter). How far this food habit contributed to better N.S. is hard to state in numerical terms; however, it is evident from the prevalent analysis in Chapter 5 that Bishnoi children are among the healthiest in the sample.
6. Singh, *Agricultural Geography*, pp. 289-93.
7. *Ibid.*, p. 264.
8. *Ibid.*, p. 278.
9. For a discussion on Ayurvedic medicine system see S.M. Bhardwaj, "Medical Pluralism and Homeopathy: A Geographic Perspective," *Social Science and Medicine* 14B (1980), 209-16.

# 7

# Summary of Conclusions and Planning Suggestions

THE magnitude of malnutrition among young children of the developing countries has increased the need for systematic understanding and planning to combat this problem. Three basic steps are thought essential in this pursuit: the assessment of the prevalence; estimating the relative importance of the causative factors embedded in the ecology of an area; and finally, finding the optimum means of affecting those determinants which prove most limiting.

The present study is an attempt, primarily of carrying out the first two steps of this planning process through an analysis of 302 young children in the critical 6-36 months age-groups. The study was carried out in 10 purposely selected villages of Haryana, an agriculturally progressive state of North India.

Anthropometric measures (weight for age) were utilized in assessing the prevalence of Protein Calorie Malnutrition (PCM) in the studied children. Jelliffe's scheme was applied in classifying children in four PCM categories. The malnutrition problem was relatively mild in Haryana children as compared to the nation as a whole. Nevertheless, one-third of the children possessed normal health and another one-third suffered from moderately severe form of PCM (PCM III and PCM IV). Older children (age 24-36 months) emerged more vulnerable to nutritional disorders.

In spatial terms the malnourishment problem varied from village to village. Better nourished children were observed where some nutrition or immunization programs (such as in

Chandi and Firozpur Namak) were available. At other places, malnutrition varied in accordance with general socio-economic and demographic conditions of the families.

The interrelated nature of causative factors was realized, and with the use of Multiple Classification Analysis (MCA) model, the relative contribution of each contributing factor was estimated. The utility of this model was realized from two facts. First, the model accepts the mixed mode of data, usual in malnutrition studies, which most multivariate models accept with limitations. Second, the critical groups needing interventions can be easily identified from the predictor category coefficients provided by the model. In other models (*e.g.*, Multiple Regression Analysis) such an advantage is not available as the category influence is not analyzed separately. With these attributes of the MCA model, we could measure the general and specific influence of the determinant influencing the nutritional status of the studied children.

According to MCA results, infection tendency of the child and income of the family emerged as the foremost determinants of malnutrition. Occupation of the head of household, birth interval, work status of mother, food group of the child, and family size also remained significant explanators in descending order of their importance.

Respiratory and gastrointestinal infections, measured by the child's disease history, remained the leading associates of malnutrition. Most infected children were found among low income families, and generally belonged to the lower castes. High infection tendencies were related to poor quality of living conditions, narrow birth interval, inaccessibility to immunization programs, and late weaning. In those villages where immunization or applied nutrition programs were available (such as Chandi) and general environmental sanitation was improved (such as Sarangwas), the infection tendencies in children remained low irrespective of their socio-economic status.

Income's effect on the N.S. was strongly felt, particularly in very poor and very rich families. The prevalence of malnutrition (PCM III and PCM IV) was more than three times greater in low income children than in their high income counterparts. Income influence was low in breast-fed children as compared to those who subsisted on weaning or regular foods. Quality of living conditions remained sub-standard in most low income families, and that possibly lead to high infection tendencies. When asked how the families would spend their anticipated higher income, more than two-thirds of the low income families opted for social and agricultural purposes (marriage, fertilizer, etc.); rather than food. The argument that increased income generally ensures better health may not be true in low income families where social needs are perceived as more important than health. Notwithstanding the significance of income in augmenting N.S. through availabilities of food, its impact in low income families is generally limited if increase in income does not synchronize with factors such as improved environmental sanitation, and adoption of family planning.

Demographic variables of family size and birth interval suggest that children in small size families (less than three children) and with moderate spacing (close to 3 years) are generally healthy. Low food availability (carbohydrate group mainly) and high infection tendencies as a result of crowding generally lead to poor nutritional status. Economic necessity in most large families triggered the milk selling practice, even though the cultural norms did not allow them to do so. The trend persisted in villages close to major urban centers and primarily within Hindu Jats. The nutritional implications of this practice were noticed in the increasing popularity of tea among such families. In general, large size families and closely spaced children were typical in lower castes, Hindu Jats, and Meo Muslims. The need for integrated family planning and nutrition programs is highly desirable, at least in the above-mentioned groups, to combat the malnutrition problem.

The dietary analysis indicated that breast-feeding provides the major protein supply in the young children, whereas a variety of *dahls* (legumes) and cereals furnish chief protein needs of the older children. The bulk of energy needs is supplied by the cereal grains such as wheat, rice, *baajra* (a kind of millet), corn, barley, and sugar (in the form of jaggery). Geographical factors usually influenced the type of cereal in north and central zone villages, whereas millets dominated in the south zone. Lipids provided an insignificant share of the total energy supply of most families, except Bishnois and Jats among whom *ghee* (clarified butter) is popular due to cultural factors. Food group available to a child depended largely on income, education of mother, and family size. Urbanization and Green Revolution influences were also observed in the declining consumption trend of milk and protein rich legumes. The popularity of tea among the young children was one of the outcomes of such influences.

Within a socio-cultural domain, work status of mother, occupation of the head of household, and caste structure (not analyzed by MCA model) emerged the important determinants of N.S. Children belonging to working mothers were more malnourished. Most such mothers belonged to scheduled castes and cultivating castes (Hindu Jats, and Ahirs) of central and south Haryana. Poor quality of living conditions, and short full breast-feeding practices[1] probably contributed to higher infections among working mothers' children. Due to the high concentration of working mothers in central and south Haryana, special efforts are needed to educate mothers in child care at least in the above areas.

Malnourishment also remained relatively high among landless laborers and small cultivators' children. Since occupational structure in Haryana is greatly associated with caste, the nutritional variations along various occupational groups were explained in relation to caste. Children belonging to scheduled castes (primarily landless laborers), artizan, and Brahmin/Vaishya (business group) were observed more malnourished, whereas more healthy children were noticed across Jat Sikh, Bishnoi (both cultivating castes) and Khatri/Arora (business) families. Differences in attitudes towards breast-feeding, weaning, food beliefs in vegetarianism and hot and cold foods possibly contributed to varying influences on the N.S. Their precise influence on the N.S. was hard to estimate due to a confounded effect of such surrogates.

The chief "target groups" of children as identified by the category coefficients of MCA analysis belonged to the following categories:

(*a*) children with very high infection tendency;
(*b*) children of very low income families;
(*c*) children belonging to small cultivators and landless laborers;

(*d*) children born within 18 months of each other;
(*e*) children of working mothers;
(*f*) children subsisting on carbohydrate foods; and
(*g*) children belonging to families with more than four children.

In general, the MCA model remained helpful in isolating the individual variable's significance in explaining the N.S. variation of the studied children. The ecological dimension of the problem became evident from the fact that malnutrition in Haryana children was related to several interrelated factors prevailing in the studied area. The spatial dimension of the problem was realized from the prevalence analysis as the mean weights of the sampled children varied significantly across the sampled villages. An indepth analysis of the determinants of malnutrition could not be possible for each village due to a small number of observations; however, correlation analysis (Table 6.3) did indicate that the malnutrition problem at a micro-level is associated with factors specific to a location. Therefore, in orchestrating a strategy to ameliorate malnutrition, both general and specific factors should be considered, depending on the scale of operation. Briefly the utility of the geo-ecological approach in the nutrition studies seems evident in precise estimation of causes of malnutrition, and identification of target areas or populations where such factors are most operative.

## PLANNING SUGGESTIONS[2]

The chief determinants of nutrition and "target groups" of children for nutritional attention have been indicated in the foregoing for the sample population in the ten villages of Haryana. Planning elaborate nutritional strategies was not within the scope of this study. Nevertheless, some suggestions can be made toward developing nutrition planning. It must be emphasized that nutrition is a very complex problem. No single academic discipline can pretend to offer all the right solutions.

At the heart of the planning process lies analysis of alternative means for achieving preselected goals. The goals, however, must be selected in reference to the available resources and the constraints upon resource mobilization. Furthermore, the goals have to be set within the framework of social, political and economic structure, and the attendant cultural value system. These fundamental aspects cannot be ignored while developing appropriate intervention strategy. Understanding of the ongoing nutrition strategies, their strengths and shortcomings, is also essential. In short-term health planning, nutritional intervention strategies especially cannot be adequately developed without intimate contextual understanding.

There is urgent need for developing a more adequate *data base* for nutrition planning. In general, the nutrition data base is derived from maternity and child welfare centers. It is important to realize that many rural mothers never take their children to these centers.

*Intensive nutrition surveys* of the present kind, covering all income groups and different areas should be conducted to assess the malnutrition problem. Such surveys should be carried out *simultaneously* in different parts of the state during different seasons. The seasonality impact, which could not be covered in this study, should be studied carefully to observe how the nutrition situation varies from one cropping season to another. Such surveys can identify the food deficit areas, and also the low food intake groups during the lean periods. A timely delivery of the food stuffs can save the aggravation of malnutrition in the affected areas and the groups at risk.

*The preventive approach* rather than curative emphasis is suggested in developing planning strategies. Supply of supplementary foods on a mass scale to make up for the nutrient deficiencies is an expensive step. At present, only a few development "blocks" have been selected for child nutrition by the state. The selection of these blocks, however, needs to be based on identification of target groups and areas such as those suggested in this study.

The nutrition programs must be organized and implemented on the basis of selected target *groups* identified for different areas, instead of developing a blanket overall curative program for the entire state. This study shows that such target groups can be identified. For effective operationalization of nutrition programs, it is imperative that *local* cultural factors and social characteristics and norms be considered by those responsible for the programs. In the northern zone of Haryana, *e.g.*, environmental sanitation of households must be emphasized in addition to the distribution of oral Vitamin A as at present. On the other hand, the children of some caste groups such as the *Bishnois* are already well nourished because of their traditional emphasis on milk and milk products. Such groups need not be required to participate fully in official supplemental food programs. A careful analysis of the variables influencing the nutritional status in different areas appears to be a prerequisite for any effective strategy to ameliorate the problem. This study shows that different clusters of factors could be responsible in different parts of the state. The need for geographic sensitivity is indicated.

Field experience in Haryana and other parts of North India shows that there are a large number of indigenous physicians in rural areas who practise various forms of traditional medicine. Frequently, these physicians are popular among the rural people. Generally, however, these traditional physicians do not have adequate knowledge of the modern concepts of nutrition. The shortage of health personnel in rural areas might be ameliorated if these indigenous physicians can be given elementary nutrition education which they can, in turn, use to improve child nutrition in the village.

*The delivery of health care* for the young children and mothers in the rural areas could be greatly improved if each primary health center is staffed with a nutrition expert who will look into the nutrition problem of his block. The author's field experience indicates that most doctors in the primary health centers have been trained in the curative methods rather than in nutrition education. It is strongly suggested that the services of the integrated child health programs be delivered at the village level rather than having the mothers and children reach the centers, which they most likely will not. In this field, there is a need for coordinated planning, *e.g.*, childhood immunization, family planning, and sanitary education. To minimize the cost of nutrition programs, resources should be allocated after a scientific assessment of the needs, applying the concept of regionalization, precise evaluation, and feedback strategies.

## REFERENCES

1. Although partial breast-feeding continues even until 30 months, the nutritional benefit of such a practice is limited as milk availability to the child is meagre a few months after birth.
2. The planning suggestions mentioned here are part of an earlier co-authored study, see S.K. Aggarwal and S.M. Bhardwaj, *Applied Medical Geography and the Developing World.*

# Appendices

## *APPENDIX A*

**Village Directory**

| Village | Physical Characteristics | | | Land Utilization, Cropping Patterns, and Irrigation (Average for 1971-72) (Area in Acres) | | | | | | |
|---|---|---|---|---|---|---|---|---|---|---|
| | Topo-graphic | Soil | Annual R.F. (hm) | Net area sown and per cent to culti-vable area | Cropped area per head of popula-tion | Per cent Cropped Area under Major Crops | | | | % irriga-tion to total cropped area |
| | | | | | | Wheat and Rice | Millets and Barley | Pulses | Commer-cial crops | |
| 1 | 2 | 3 | 4 | 5 | 6 | 7 | 8 | 9 | 10 | 11 |
| *North Zone Villages* | | | | | | | | | | |
| Manakpur | Piedmont | Piedmont | 1000-1100 | 454 (94.2) | 0.63 | 96 (14.5) | 128 (19.3) | 206 (31.1) | 157 (23.7) | 9 (1.4) |
| Mehra | Alluvial Plain | Silt/Clay | 700-800 | 660 (97.6) | 0.53 | 426 (52.1) | 108 (13.2) | 48 (5.8) | 181 (22.1) | 755 (92.4) |
| Sangatpura | Alluvial Plain | Loam | 400-500 | 439 (98.7) | 0.38 | 48 (9.3) | 275 (53.5) | 78 (15.2) | 38 (7.4) | 224 (43.6) |

| 1 | 2 | 3 | 4 | 5 | 6 | 7 | 8 | 9 | 10 | 11 |
|---|---|---|---|---|---|---|---|---|---|---|
| *Central Zone Villages* | | | | | | | | | | |
| Salamkhera | Flood Plain | Sandy Soft Loam | 300-400 | 1028 (92.4) | 1.50 | 142 (13.1) | 88 (8.1) | 449 (41.5) | 190 (16.6) | 416 (38.5) |
| Landheri | Alluvial Plain (Sandy) | Sandy Loam | 300-400 | 1206 (87.1) | 0.56 | 139 (8.0) | 197 (11.3) | 385 (22.1) | 721 (41.4) | 1280 (73.4) |
| Chandi | Alluvial Plain | Loam | 500-600 | 2131 (95.9) | 0.80 | 428 (14.9) | 1027 (35.6) | 604 (20.9) | 271 (9.5) | 1854 (64.3) |
| *South Zone Villages* | | | | | | | | | | |
| Pirthala | Alluvial Plain | Sandy Loam | 500-600 | 1125 (99.7) | 0.37 | 340 (26.5) | 382 (29.8) | 186 (14.5) | 50 (3.9) | 271 (21.1) |
| Firozpur Namak | Hilly and Alluvial | Coarse Loam | 500-600 | 315 (1.00) | 0.24 | 19 (4.1) | 181 (38.8) | 198 (42.4) | 26 (5.6) | 12 (2.6) |
| Sarangwas | Sand Dunes | Sandy | 400-500 | 985 (93.5) | 1.00 | 2 (0.1) | 758 (40.4) | 862 (45.9) | 4 (0.2) | 3 (0.2) |
| Rajgarh | Undulating Sandy Plain | Light Loam | 300-400 | 138 (93.2) | 0.12 | 37 (19.7) | 66 (35.1) | 13 (6.9) | 19 (10.1) | 57 (30.3) |

*(Contd.)*

APPENDIX A (*Contd.*)

| | Population Characteristics | | Amenities Available (Distance in Kilometers) | | | | |
|---|---|---|---|---|---|---|---|
| | Major Castes | Total Population | Educational | Marketing Facility | Medical Facility | Bus Stop | Drinking Water Facility |
| | 12 | 13 | 14 | 15 | 16 | 17 | 18 |
| *North Zone Villages* | | | | | | | |
| Manakpur | Khatri, Arora, Brahmin, Scheduled Castes | 1048 | P.M. | 3 | 3 | 2 | HP, Well |
| Mehra | Hindu Jats, Scheduled Caste Jat Sikh, Artizan | 1517 | P | 4 | 4 | 3 | HP, W |
| Sangatpura | Jat, Scheduled Caste | 1337 | P | 5 | 5 | 6 | W |
| *Central Zone Villages* | | | | | | | |
| Salamkhera | Scheduled Castes, Jats, Jat Sikh, Khatri, Arora | 721 | P | 12 | 2 | 2 | Pipe, C |

| | 12 | 13 | 14 | 15 | 16 | 17 | 18 |
|---|---|---|---|---|---|---|---|
| Landheri | Bishnoi, Rajput, Brahmin, Scheduled Castes | 3070 | H | 22 | 20 | 0 | HP, W |
| Chandi | Arora, Jats, Scheduled Castes | 3463 | H | 3 | 3 | 0 | HP, W |
| *South Zone Villages* | | | | | | | |
| Pirthala | Jat, Brahmin, Bania, Scheduled Castes | 3491 | H | 11 | 0 | 0 | HP, Pipe |
| Firozpur Namak | Meo, Scheduled Castes | 1939 | P | 3 | 0 | 0 | Pipe |
| Sarangwas | Ahirs, Brahmin, Scheduled Castes | 1833 | P | 13 | 3 | 3 | Pipe |
| Rajgarh | Rajput, Ahirs, Scheduled Castes | 1473 | P | 3 | 3 | 0 | Pipe, Well |

HP — Hand Pump
W — Open Well
P — Primary School
M — Middle School
H — High School
C — Canal

## *APPENDIX B*

## The Questionnaire

Card Serial Number ..........................................................
Subject Identity Number ..................................................
Date of Interview: (Day, Month, Year)

**Anthropometric Information on the Child**

(1) Sex: Male: 1 Female: 2
(2) Age (months)
(3) Weight (kg.)
(4) Height (cms.)

**Socio-Economic Information on the Household**

Social Factors
Occupation of the Head of Household

| | |
|---|---|
| Cultivators | |
| Less than 10 acres | 1 |
| 11-30 acres | 2 |
| 30 and above | 3 |
| Business and Commerce | |
| Professional | |
| Service (Clerk, etc.) | 4 |
| Landless laborer | 5 |

Social Status (Caste)..........................................................
Family Structure

| | |
|---|---|
| Nuclear Single | 1 |
| Joint | 2 |

Total number of persons living in the Family......................
(if joint)
Education in the Family

| | |
|---|---|
| Father : Not literate | 1 |
| Elementary— middle | 2 |
| High School | 3 |
| Beyond High School | 4 |

Mother : Not literate 1
Elementary—middle 2
High School 3
Beyond High School 4

Economic Factors

Family annual income from all sources:

| | |
|---|---|
| Rs. 0-1200 | 1 |
| 1201-2400 | 2 |
| 2401-4800 | 3 |
| 4801-8400 | 4 |
| 8401 and above | 5 |

Proportion of income spent on food:

| | |
|---|---|
| One-third | 1 |
| One-half | 2 |
| Two-thirds | 3 |
| More than two-thirds | 4 |

If there is an increase in your income, will you spend it for your child's food or for some other purposes?

Child............................ Other purpose..........................
For both..........................

**Information on Cultural Influences of Dietary Intake**

What is your religion?

| | | | |
|---|---|---|---|
| Hinduism | 1 | Islam | 4 |
| Sikhism | 2 | Jainism | 5 |
| Christianity | 3 | Others | 6 |

Food Attitudes

| | |
|---|---|
| Vegetarian by choice | 1 |
| Non-vegetarian | 2 |
| Not strict vegetarian | 3 |

Do you believe that some foods are of hot and cold nature and you should not give it to your child?

Yes 1 No 2

If yes, name some of such foods:

| Hot foods | Cold foods |
|---|---|
| ........................ | ........................ |
| ........................ | ........................ |
| ........................ | ........................ |
| ........................ | ........................ |

Do you fear you will be ostracized if your child starts using some nutritious food (*e.g.*, meat, egg, etc.), which otherwise is not permissible in your caste?

Yes 1 No 2

Modernity Factors

What practice do/did you use in feeding milk to the child?

Breast-feeding (1) Both (3)
Bottle-feeding (2)

At what age was this child weaned or should be weaned?

| | |
|---|---|
| Six months | 1 |
| One year | 2 |
| More than one year | 3 |

Method of stopping breast-feeding

| | |
|---|---|
| Abrupt | 1 |
| Gradual | 2 |

Where do you generally take your child for minor health problems (such as diarrhea, fever, cough)?

| | |
|---|---|
| Physician (Angrezi Doctor) | 1 |
| Village Doctor (Vaidya, Hakim) | 2 |
| Magic/Witchcraft/Siana | 3 |
| Homeopath | 4 |

Total number of persons in the family..............................

Average spacing of children (up to 10 years of age):

| | |
|---|---|
| Less than 18 months | 1 |
| 19-36 months | 2 |
| More than 36 months | 3 |
| Only child | 4 |

Do you practice family planning methods?

Yes 1 No 2

Do you sell milk/butter/poultry for economic reasons?

Yes 1 No 2

Food crops available for consumption

1. ........................
2. ........................
3. ........................

Did you get your child immunized to the following diseases?

| | | |
|---|---|---|
| Polio | : Yes 1 | No 2 |
| Cholera | : Yes 1 | No 2 |
| Small Pox | : Yes 1 | No 2 |
| Typhoid | : Yes 1 | No 2 |

How often does the child fall sick?
(Diarrhea, Fever, Cough, etc.)

| | | |
|---|---|---|
| Diarrhea | : Frequently 1 | Infrequently 2 |
| Cough | : Frequently 1 | Infrequently 2 |
| Fever | : Frequently 1 | Infrequently 2 |

Infection tendency:

Low 1 Moderate 2 High 3

Do you wash your hands before cooking or feeding the child?

Often 1 Sometimes 2 Generally not 3

Where do you take your child when he is sick?
Government Dispensary/Doctor/Siana/Hakim/Vaidya
Name of the place..........................................................
Distance from home..................................miles

**Micro Environment (to be evaluated by the investigation)**

Predominant source of water for drinking:

| | | | |
|---|---|---|---|
| Hand Pump/Tube Well | 1 | Canal | 4 |
| Well | 2 | Others | 5 |
| Baori | 3 | | |

Quality of the house (assessed in terms of floor, walls, maintenance, building material, rubbish disposal, density of rooms, sanitary conditions):

| | |
|---|---|
| Very good | 1 |
| Satisfactory | 2 |
| Poor | 3 |

Air circulation and sunlight in the living rooms:

| | |
|---|---|
| Very good | 1 |
| Satisfactory | 2 |
| Poor | 3 |

Cleanliness of the child:

| | |
|---|---|
| Very good | 1 |
| Satisfactory | 2 |
| Poor | 3 |

Condition of cooking utensils:

| | |
|---|---|
| Very good | 1 |
| Satisfactory | 2 |
| Poor | 3 |

# Bibliography

Aggarwal, S.K., and S.M. Bhardwaj, "Applied Medical Geography and the Developing World: With a Case Study of Malnutrition," in *Applied Geography: Selected Perspectives*, ed. Frazier, J.W. Englewood Cliffs: N.J.: Prentice Hall, 1982.

American Institute of Nutrition and American Medical Association, *Proceedings of Third Western Hemisphere Nutrition Congress,* Mount Kisco, New York: Futura Publishing Company, 1972.

Andrews, Frank M., James N. Morgan, John A. Sonquist, and Laura Klem, *Multiple Classification Analysis*, Ann Arbor, Michigan: The University of Michigan, 1975.

Andrews, S., *Feasibility of Involving Indigenous Medical Practitioners For Family Planning Services Delivery in Kerala, India*, Ph.D. Dissertation, John Hopkins University, 1973.

Arnold, R., "The Quack Stick: A Field Measure Used by The Quaker Service Team, Nigeria," 1969, Nigeria, *J. Trop. Pediat.* 15 (1969).

Austin, James E., and James F. Levinson, "Population and Nutrition: A Case Study for Integration," Milbank *Memorial Fund Quarterly*, 52 (1974), 169-84.

Aykrod, W.R., "Conquest of Deficiency Diseases: Protein-Calorie-Malnutrition," *Indian Journal of Medical Science*, 25, (1971), 415-430.

Azad, R.N., "Nutrition In The Context of Food Shortage And Rising Population," *Kurukshetra*, 23 (February 1975), 11-13.

Banik, N.D., Datta, R. Krishna, S.I.S. Mane, and Lila Raj, "A Longitudinal Study of Protein Calorie Malnutrition In North Indian Pre-School Children," *Indian Journal of Pediatrics*, 38 (1971), 147-52.

Banik, N.D., S. Nayar, R. Krishna, L. Raj, "A Study of Epidemiologic Basis of Malnutrition in Pre-School Children

In Slum Areas in Delhi," *Indian Pediatrics*, 10 (January 1973), 25.

Bengoa, T.M., "The Problem of Malnutrition", *WHO Chronicle*, 28 (1974), 3-7.

Berg, Alan, *The Nutrition Factor: Its Role In National Development*, Washington, D.C.: The Brookings Institution, 1973.

Berg, A., Nevin S. Scrimshaw, and David L. Call, *Nutrition, National Development and Planning*, Cambridge: The M.I.T. Press, 1973.

Berg, Alan, and Robert Muscat, "Nutrition Program Planning: An Approach," in *Nutrition, National Development and Planning*, pp. 247-74, Edited by Alan Berg, Nevin S. Scrimshaw, David L. Call, Cambridge: The M.I.T. Press, 1973.

Berrien, F. Kenneth, *General and Social Systems*, New Jersey: Rutgers University Press, 1968.

Bertaslanfey, Von, *General Systems Theory*, New York: George Bra-Zillar, 1968.

Bhalla, G.S., *Changing Agrarian Structure in India*, Delhi: Meenakshi Prakashan, 1974.

Bhandari, B., A.M. Jain, Padma Karna, Asha Mathur, and V.K. Sharma, "Nutritional Anthropometry of Rural School Children of Udaipur District," *Indian Journal of Pediatrics*, 39 (January 1972), 1-11.

Bhardari, N.R., and G.P. Pateel, "Dietary and Feeding Habits of Infants in Various Socio-Economic Groups," *Indian Pediatrics*, 10 (April 1973), 233-38.

Bhardwaj, S.M, "Medical Pluralism and Homeopathy: A geographic Perspective," *Social Science and Medicine*, 14B (1980), 209-16.

Blyn, George, "Nutritional Adequacy of Punjab and Haryana Cultivator Families," Paper presented at the *Sixth Annual Wisconsin Conference* on South Asia, University of Wisconsin-Madison, November 6, 1977.

Call, David L. and F. James Levinson, "A Systematic Approach to Nutrition Intervention Programs." In *Nutrition, National Development and Planning*, pp. 165-97, Edited by Alan Berg, Nevin S. Scrimshaw, David L. Call, Cambridge: The M.I.T. Press, 1973.

Chafkin, Sol., *An Operations Oriented Study of Nutrition as an Integrated System of Tamilnadu* (Report prepared for Food and Nutrition Division, U.S. Agency for International Development, New Delhi, Feburary 11, 1970).

Chakravarti, A.K., "Regional Preferences for Food: Some Aspects of Food Habit Patterns in India," *Canadian Geographer*, 18 (1974), 395-410.

Chatterjee, G.C., "Nutritional Problems of India," *Science and Culture*, 42 (1976), 3-7.

Chauduri, M.K., "Nutritional Profile of Calcutta Pre-School Children, II, Clinical Observations", *Indian Journal of Medical Research*, 62 (February 1975), 189-95.

Chib, Sukhdev Singh, *This Beautiful India: Haryana*, New Delhi: Light & Life Publishers, 1977.

Chikermane, A.S., "Socio-Cultural and Economic Aspects of Infant Feeding and Malnutrition", *Indian Pediatrics*, 12 (January 1975), 20-21.

Chroley, R.J., "Geography As Human Ecology," in *Directions in Geography*, pp. 155-70, Edited by Richard J. Chroley, London: Methuen & Company, 1973.

Deodhor, N.S., "Social and Cultural Factors Conditioning Infant Feeding," *Indian Journal of Medical Science*, 21 (November 1967), 770-972.

Devdas, Rajmal P., "Social and Cultural Factors Influencing Malnutrition," *Journal of Home Economics*, 62 (March 1973), 164-71.

Ghai, O.P., and Vimlish Seth, "Grading of Protein Calorie Malnutrition," *Indian Pediatrics*, 9 (December 1972), 727-31.

Ghai, O.P., "Feeding Habits in Relation to Diarrhea and Malnutrition," *Indian Pediatrics*, 12 (1975).

Ghai, O.P., "Assessment of Protein Calorie Malnutrition", *Indian Pediatrics*, 12 (1975).

Girt, John L., "The Geography of Non-Vectored Infectious Diseases," In John M. Hunter, ed. *Geography of Health and Disease*, pp. 81-100, Chapel Hill: Department of Geography, University of North Carolina, 1974.

Golikere, R.K., *Vegetarianism vs Non-vegetarianism*, Bombay: Popular Books, 1960.

Gopalan, C., "Studies on Lactation in Poor Indian Communities," *Journal of Tropical Pediatrics* (December 1958), 92.

Gopalan, C., Presidential Address, *Proceedings of the First Asian Congress on Nutrition*, Hyderabad, India, 1972.

Gopalan, C., S.C. Balasubramaniam, B.V. Rama Sastri, and Visweswara Rao, *Diet Atlas of India*, Hyderabad: National Institute of Nutrition, 1971.

Gopalan, C., and B.S. Narsingha Rao, "Nutritional Constraints on Growth and Development in Current Indian Dietaries," *Indian Journal of Medical Research*, 59 (June 1971), 111-21.

Gopalan, C., and K. Vijaya Raghavan, *Nutrition Atlas of India*, Hyderabad: National Institute of Nutrition, Indian Council of Medical Research, 1971.

Gopalan, C., and Nandamuni Naidu, "Nutrition and Fertility," Lancet (November 18, 1972), 1077-79.

Government of India, *Report of the Health Survey and Planning Committee*, New Delhi: Government of India Press, 1972.

Government of India, Planning Commission, *Draft Fifth Five Year Plan: 1974-79*, Vol. II, New Delhi: Government of India Press, 1973.

Government of India, *Fourth Five Year Plan*, New Delhi: Government of India Publication, 1973.

Gyorgy, Paul, and O.L. Kline, ed. *Malnutrition is a Problem of Ecology*, New York: Karger, 1970.

Heer, D.M., and D.O. Smith, "Mortality Level, Desired Family Size, and Population Increase," *Demography*, 5 (1968), 104-21.

Husain, S. Sajid, "Nutritional Deficiency Diseases in Badaun and Shahjahanpur Districts", *The Geographer*, 16 (1967), 45-56.

Indian Council of Medical Research, and Indian Council of Social Research, *Alternative Approaches to the Health Care*, New Delhi: Indian Council of Medical Research, c. 1977.

Jelliffe, E.F.P., and M. Gurney, "Definition of the Problem," pp. 1-14, In Alex F. Roche and Frank Falknew, *Nutrition and Malnutrition: Identification and Measurement*, London and New York: Plenum Press, 1974.

Jelliffee, D.B., *The Assessment of the Nutritional Status of the Community*, Geneva: World Health Organization, 1966.

John Hopkins University, *Functional Analysis of Health Needs and Services*, mimeographed, Baltimore: Department of International Health, John Hopkins University, 1970.

Kanawati, A.A., and D.S. McLaren, "Mid-Arm/Head Circumference Ratio: A New Technique to Assess Marginal Protein-Calorie Malnutrition in a Community." In *Proceedings of the First Asian Congress on Nutrition*, 786-89, Hyderabad, India, 1972.

Khan, Zahoor Ali, "Nutritional Deficiency Disease and Environmental Factors in the Central Ganga-Yamuna Doab," *The Geographers*, 16 (1969), 57-77, 1969.

Khanna, K.K., "Nutrition and Population," *Indian Pediatrics*, 8 (1971), 217-18, 1971.

Knight, C., Gregary and R. Paul Wilcox, *Triumph or Triage: The World Food Problem in Geographical Perspective*, AAG Resource Paper, 75-3, Washington, D.C.: Association of American Geographers, 1976.

Kumar, Ajit, Y.C. Mathur, and Harish Chander, "A Study of the Morbidity Pattern Amongst Pre-School Children in a Rural Area," *Indian Pediatrics*, 9 (1973), 327-31, 1972.

Lal, Muni, *Haryana on High Road to Prosperity*, Delhi: Vikas Publishing House, 1974.

Laszlo, Ervin, *Introduction to Systems Philosophy*, New York: Harper and Row Publishers, 1972.

Levinson, F. James, *Morinda: An Economic Analysis of Malnutrition Among Young Children in Rural India*, Cornell-MIT International Nutrition Policy Series, Vol. I, Cambridge, Mass., 1974.

Loewenstein, Mathew S., and James F. Phillips, "Evaluation of Arm Circumference Measurement for Determining Nutritional Status of Children and Its Use in an Acute Epidemic of Malnutrition: Owerri, Nigeria, Following the Nigerian Civil War," *The American Journal of Clinical Nutrition*, 26 (February 1973), 226-33.

Mathur, J.S., S.K. Mehrotra, and B.B. Maheshwari, "Nutritional Disorders Among Children Below 5 years in a Rural Community," *Indian Journal of Pediatrics*, 41 (1974), 185-91.

May, Jacques M., "Medical Geography: Its Methods and Objectives," *Geographical Review*, 40 (1950), 9-41.

May, Jacques M., *The Ecology of Human Disease*, New York: MD Publications, Inc., 1958.

McLaren, D.S., and P.L. Pell, "Nutrition in the Middle East", In *World Review of Nutrition and Dietetics*, 12, 43-127, New York: Karger, 1970.

Miller, D.S., and P.R. Payne, "Assessment of Protein Requirements," *Proc. Nutr. Soc.* 28 (1969), 225.

Narangwal Rural Health Research, "Interaction of Nutrition and Infection Study," In *Village Nutrition Studies: An Annotated Bibliography*, pp. 129-30, Eds. Sue, Schofield, and C.M. Lambart, Sussex: Institute of Development Studies, University of Sussex, 1969.

Newman, James E., and Robert C. Pickett, "World Climates and Food Supply Variations," *Science*, 186 (December 6, 1974), 877-81.

Osima, Harry T., "Food Consumption, Nutrition and Economic Development," *Economic Development and Cultural Change*, 15 (1967), 385-97.

Pant, Pitambar, "Food, Nutrition, Population and Economic Development," In *Proceedings of the First Asian Congress of Nutrition*, pp. 286-309, Edited by P.G. Tulpule and Kamla S. Jayanti Rao, Hyderabad: National Institute on Nutrition, 1972.

Patwardhan, V.N., "Geographic Distribution of Malnutrition", In *Proceedings of the Seventh International Congress of Nutrition*, Vol. 1, pp. 27-33, Toronto: Pergamon Press, 1966.

Pereria, S.M., "Growth and Development of Children in Under Privileged Communities, Tamilnadu," *Indian Journal of Medical Research*, 59 (June 1971), 164-76.

Planalp, T.M., *Heat Stress and Culture in North India*, Natick, Mass: U.S. Army Research Institute, 1971.

Pollack, Herbert, Geographic Peculiarities of Nutrition," In *Proceedings of the Seventh International Congress of Nutrition*, Vol. 1, pp. 362-80, Toronto: Pergamon Press, 1966.

Prakash, Budha, *Haryana Through The Ages*, Kurukshetra, India, Kurukshetra University Press, 1970.

Rao, T.M.V., J. Gourinath Sastri, and K. Vijay Raghavan, "Nutritional Status of Children in Urban Slums Around Delhi," *Indian Journal of Medical Research* (October 1974), 1492-98.

Rathor, B.S., H.S. Mathur, and S. Saxena, "Nutritional Anthropometry of 100 Children Dwelling in Slum Areas of Jaipur Compared to that of 500 Children of the Elite". *Indian Journal of Pediatrics*, 42 (September 1977), 264-76.

Robinow, Meihard, and D.B. Jelliff, "Intercorrelations Between Anthropometric Variables, A Contribution to Nutrition Anthropometry of Infancy and Early Childhood in Developing Countries," *Proceedings of the Seventh International Congress of Nutrition*, Vol. 4, 144-47, Hamburg, Toronto: Pergamon Press.

Roy, P., "The Sacred Cow in India", *Rural Sociology*, 20, (1955), 8-15.

Sanjur, D., and E. Romero, "Conceptual Levels of Dietary Indicators as Predictors of Nutritional Status," *Nutrition*, 2 (1975): 214-222.

Schofield, Sue Comp., and C.M. Lambert, eds. *Village Nutrition Studies*: *An Annotated Bibliography*, Sussex: Institute of Development Studies, University of Sussex, 1975.

Scrimshaw, Nevin S., "Malnutrition, Learning, and Behavior," *American Journal of Clinical Nutrition*, 20 (May 1967), 493-502.

Scrimshaw, Nevin S., Carl E. Taylor, and John E. Gordon, *Interaction of Nutrition and Infection*, Geneva: World Health Organization, 1968.

Scrimshaw, Nevin S., "Synergism of Malnutrition and Infection: Evidence From Field Studies in Guatemala," *Journal of American Medical Association*, 212 (1970), 1685-92.

Schwartzberg, Joseph E., "The Distribution of Selected Castes in the North Indian Plain," *The Geographical Review*, 55 (1965), pp. 477-96.

Sharma, S.C., "Land Use and Nutrition in the Village Manikpur in the Central Upland of the Lower Yamuna-Chambal Doab," *The Geographical Review of India*, 34 (1972), 369-85.

Simm, S.R., F. Cesario, I.L. Kline, and D.M. Yates, *A Systems Approach to the World Protein Problem*, Report prepared by the Battelle Memorial Institute for the United Nations Protein Advisory Group, May 6, 1970.

Singh, Jasbir, *An Agricultural Geography of Haryana*, Kurukshetra, India: Vishal Publications, 1976.

Stoddart, D.R., "Geography and the Ecological Approach," *Geography*, 50 (1965), 242-51.

Sukhatme, P.V., 1970, "Protein Deficiency in Urban and Rural Areas," *Proceedings of the Nutrition Society*, (London) 29 (May 1970), 176-83.

Wilson, C.S., Food Habits: A Selected Annotated Bibliography, *Journal of Nutritional Education*, (Supplement, 1973).

World Bank, *Health*, Sector Policy Paper March 1975, 80.

World Health Organization, Joint FAO/UNICEF/WHO Expert Committee Report, *Methodology of Nutritional Surveillance*, WHO Tech. Rep. Ser., No. 593, Geneva: World Health Organization, 1976.

World Health Organization, *World Health Statistics Report*, Vol. 26, No. 11, 1973, Sec. II.

Wyon, John B., and John E. Gordon, *The Khanna Study: Population Problems in the Rural Punjab*, Cambridge: Harvard University Press, 1971.

# Index

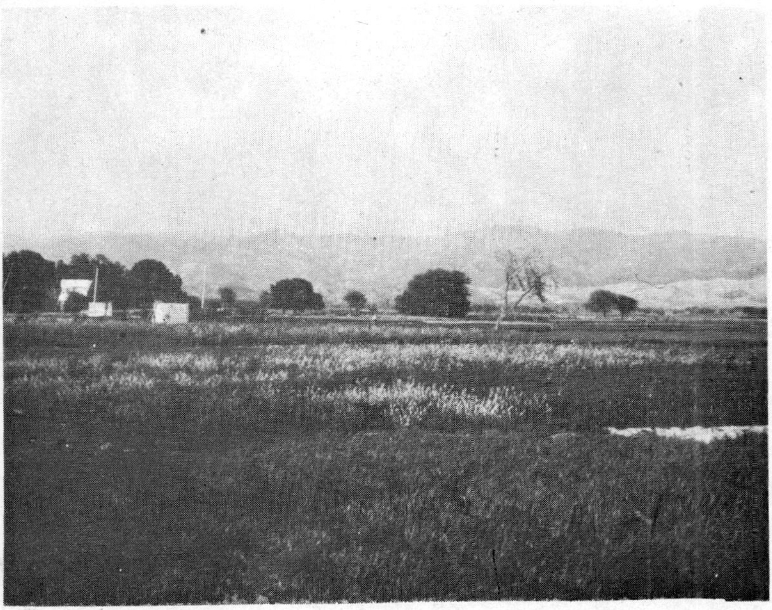

1. Northern part of the North region contains hilly and undulating terrain with poor soils. Wherever regular irrigation facilities are available, agricultural productivity brings prosperity to the area and hence better nutritional standards.

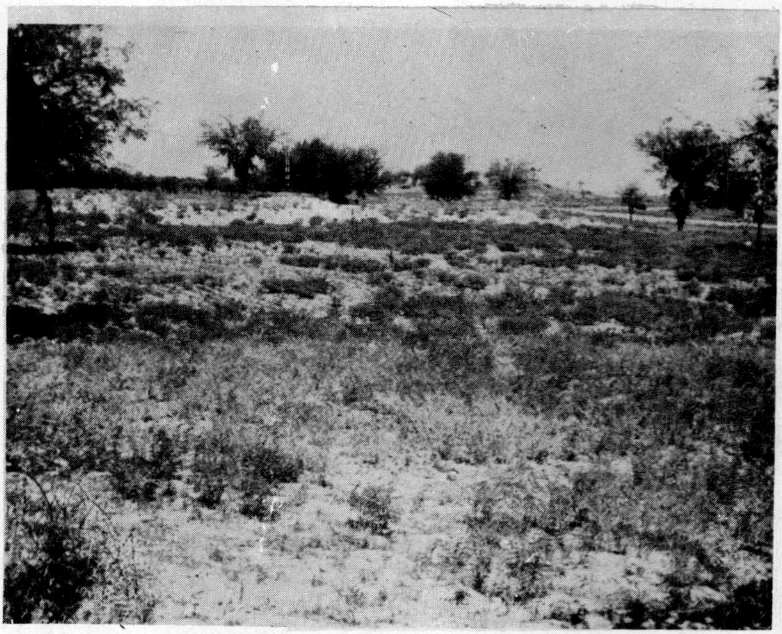

2. The southern part of Haryana is typical of sandy soils and outliers of the Aravalli hills. Poor soils and rough terrain keep the agricultural productivity low and so are the nutritional intakes.

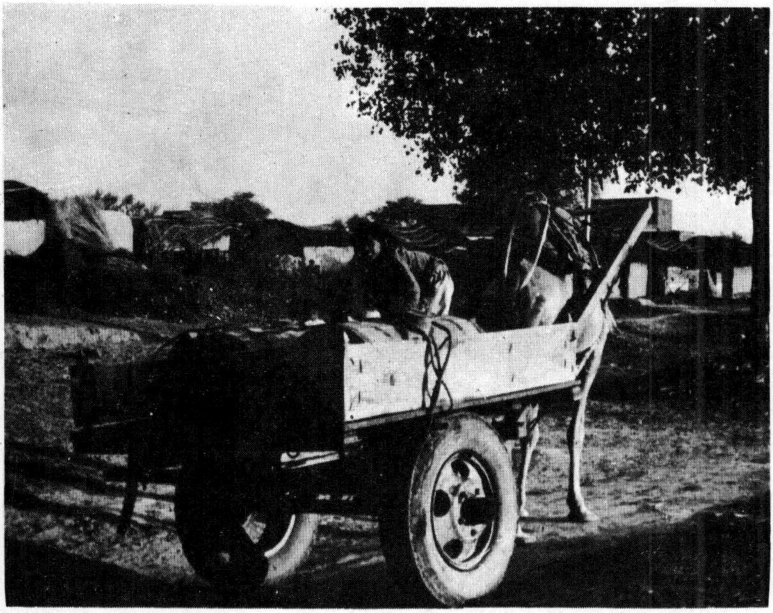

3. Wherever regular water supply is made available through government efforts water-borne diseases are of less magnitude and nutritional status is found better irrespective of income levels.

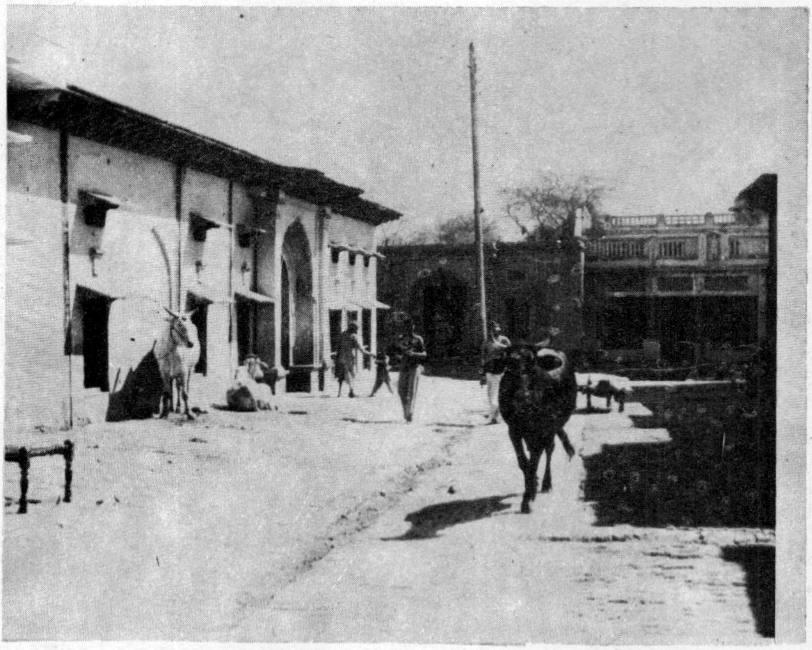

4. Residential quarters of the high-income Bishnoi farmers present better living conditions. The Bishnoi farmers greatly emphasize the consumption of milk and milk products by their families. The children are usually well nourished.

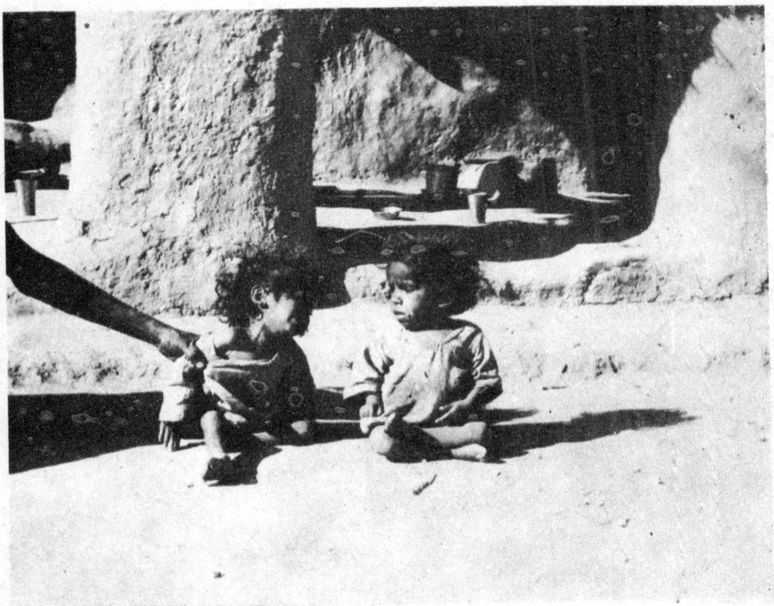

5. Severe protein-energy malnutrition is characteristic of the very poor families. These twin sisters show several obvious signs of malnutrition.

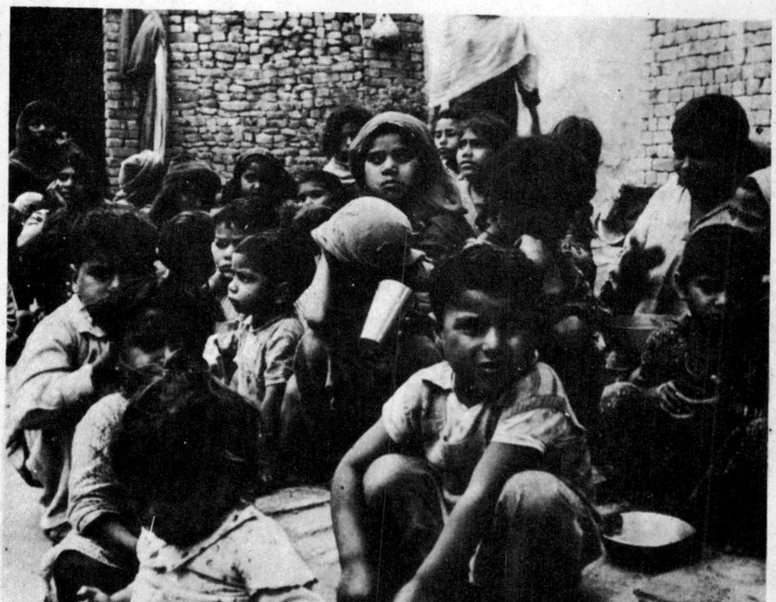

6. Well planned supplementary feeding programmes can have remarkable impact on the health of rural children.

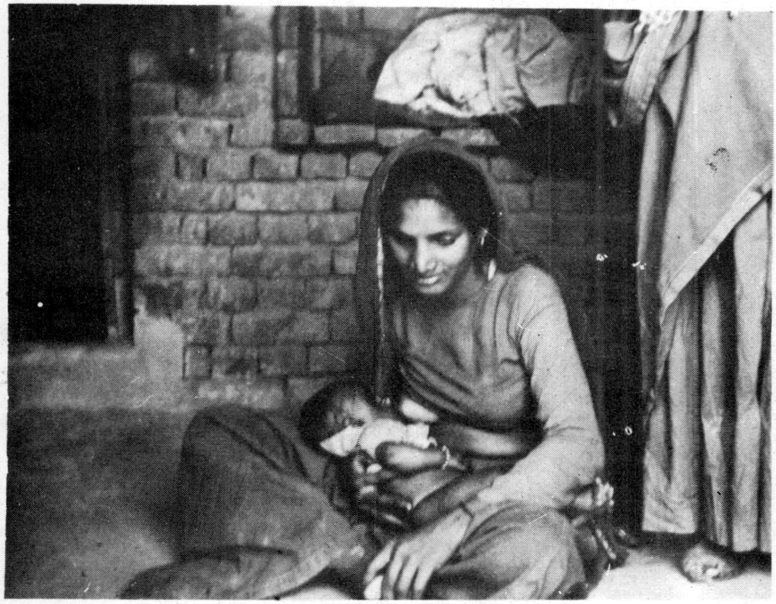

7. Breast feeding is common in Haryana. This probably accounts for low incidence of protein-energy malnutrition among children during the first twelve months of age.

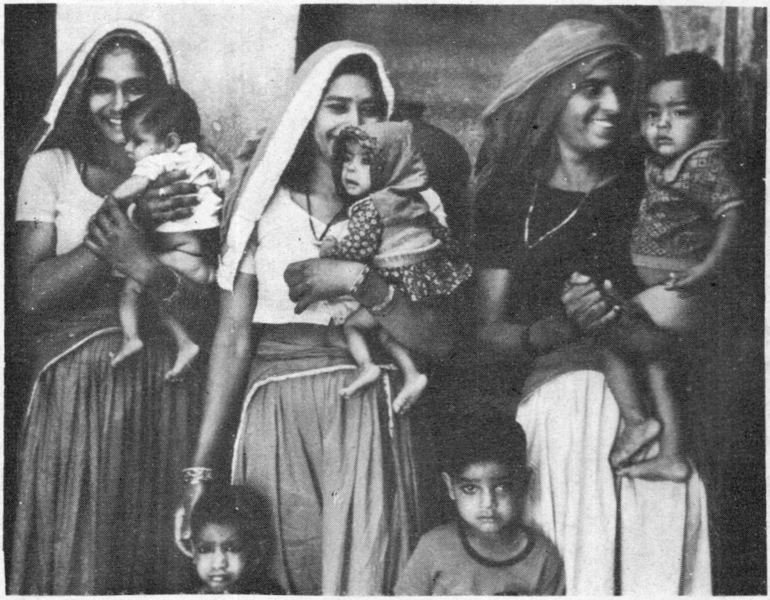

8. Children living in the joint family system are sometimes better nourished due to the extra care available, if the mother has to attend to the farming operations.